ADV.

"[The authors] are from diverse backgrounds but united in their spiritual strength and their faith in meeting the challenge of dealing with cancer. They have navigated a very difficult path, learning that life is a gift and should be celebrated, not wasted. Even after the first few stories, I was amazed by how true the stories were, and by how the authors have laid bare their fears, emotional upheavals, and stresses that may have led to their illness. Each author has written in a conversational style, sharing their failings, their recognition of the trials ahead, and their determination to not let life browbeat them. Having emotional, mental, and spiritual support, along with appropriate professional intervention, can put up a fight against [the challenge of cancer]. This book is a big support. Each author is not only a Cancer Hero but a Champion of Life, helping others by sharing her personal journey and, in doing so, inspiring readers to find their own strength and faith to not give up."
— *Dr. Rati Vajpey, HOM (Can), MD (Ind), FISC (UK), CAN Coach (Can), Clinical Oncologist*

"I understand that receiving a cancer diagnosis or caring for a loved one with cancer can be an incredibly difficult and emotional experience. It is natural to feel overwhelmed and hopeless at times. However, I genuinely believe that this book can offer a source of comfort and hope for those who are going through this challenging journey. It can remind them that they are not alone in their struggles and that there is a community of people who have faced similar challenges and come out stronger."
—*Dr. Iman Taheri, Iranian-Canadian Surgeon, Philanthropist, and Poet*

CANCER HEROES

*Lovingly Woven Stories of Healing, Survival
& Profound Transformation*

Curated by Shirin Ariff

With authentic cancer stories written by
Shirin Ariff, Pat Labez, CoCo Roper, LaCountess R. Ingram,
Rowena Rodriguez, Shirley Gaudon, Niki Papaioannou, Tania
Kolar, and Catherine Clark

With Foreword by Peggy McColl

Paperback: 978-1-7381171-0-9
eBook: 978-1-7381171-1-6

First Paperback Edition: February 2024

Printed in the USA
1 2 3 4 5 6 7 8 9 10

ENTOURAGE

Published by Entourage Media & Marketing Inc.
www.entouragemedia.ca

First and foremost, for my Aunt Sultana Tikari,
who passed away after an honorable journey with cancer.
And for all those who seek hope as they embark on their own cancer
journey or reflect upon the milestones and resting points
of a life well-lived.

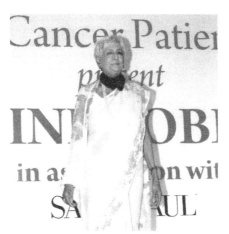

Sultana Tikari

CONTENTS

Cancer Heroes are all around us.
They are the survivors who offer hope to all they encounter,
the nurturers who hold their best friend's hand during
chemotherapy, and the beautiful souls who leave a legacy of impact
that rings just as loud as any remission bell.

DISCLAIMER

This book is not intended to promote, prescribe, or recommend any specific cancer treatment or alternative healing modality and/or any religious views. The expressed opinions of the authors are based on their own lived experiences. It is recommended that you seek the advice and support of trusted professionals.

CANCER HEROES

FOREWORD

by Peggy McColl

In the pages that follow, you will find stories that are more than just narratives; they are beacons of light in the darkest of times. "Cancer Heroes" is not merely a title but an embodiment of courage, an anthology of battles where the human spirit shines brightest against the shadow of adversity.

As someone who has intimately known the precipice between health and illness, I have come to understand that the term "survivor" barely scratches the surface of the journey one undertakes when faced with cancer. My own path through metastatic cancer was not just about surviving. It was about transcending. It was about the alchemy of turning fear into fortitude, pain into purpose, and illness into insight.

These lovingly woven stories are testimonials to an undeniable truth that I have seen echoed in every facet of personal development and success since I first embarked on this path in 1979. We hold within us the extraordinary ability to transform our lives. We are creators, architects of our own miracles, and masters of our destinies.

As a New York Times bestselling author, with over two decades dedicated to teaching the principles of manifestation and success, I can attest to the power of the human mind and spirit to initiate profound change. What defines a hero is not merely the victory, but the journey undertaken and the growth that occurs within.

The individuals you will meet in this book have not just faced their battles with cancer; they have embraced transformation in its most profound sense. Their stories are not just about survival—they are about a transcendence that inspires a renaissance of the self, manifesting new beginnings and possibilities.

As you turn each page, allow these stories to serve as a mirror, reflecting the boundless resilience that resides within you. May you find comfort in the shared experiences, strength in the collective wisdom, and, above all, a renewed belief in the possibility of healing and transformation that awaits us all.

We are all heroes in our own stories, and this book is a celebration of that indomitable spirit. Welcome to a journey of healing, survival, and profound transformation. Welcome to the chronicles of the truest heroes among us.

With warmest regards and heartfelt solidarity,

Peggy McColl, New York Times Bestselling Author and Manifestation Mentor
www.PeggyMcColl.com

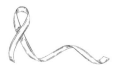

PROLOGUE

by Shirin Ariff

This book serves as a heartfelt tribute to all my family members who lost their battles with cancer. It is also an expression of deep admiration for those who survived this killer disease. Above all, it is dedicated to my beloved Aunt Sultana Tikari, who lived a full life as a cancer survivor. Despite losing her voice, she never lost her zest for life.

Anyone who witnessed her vibrant youth and then saw me would claim that I was her daughter. Many people often remark on our striking resemblance, and I take great pride in that. She was one of my favorite aunts among the four on my father's side. Out of the four, she was the only one who enjoyed good physical and mental health. Two of my aunts were born with physical disabilities, and one of them, Aunty Sakina, lost her battle with breast cancer. The third aunt suffered from mental health issues. Aunty Sultana was married to an Indian prince from the distinguished Tikari family of Bihar, India.

Whenever Aunty Sultana would visit us, I would abandon everything and rush to her side. I would stick to her like glue because I cherished every moment spent with her and couldn't bear to be anywhere else. My time with her was precious, and I didn't want to miss a single second. I adored her not just for her talents—she was renowned for her beautiful knitting and crocheting—but also for her profound love for her family. She was the nourishing foundation upon which her husband and daughter flourished. Her family knew they could always count on her. She stood shoulder to shoulder with her two younger brothers, my father and uncle, supporting the family during the darkest times. She ventured into the workforce at a time when the women in our family could never think of doing so. She was ahead of her time, and in my eyes, she was the epitome of a devoted wife and mother. She was my hero. She loved my dad, and she was always there for me. I could count on her to be by my side at the hospital during surgeries and when I gave birth to my first child. She would wait outside the operating room with my dad until she received news that everything went well and that I was safe. She would visit me in the hospital. My life mattered to her.

Aunty Sultana possessed a remarkable entrepreneurial spirit and was a master at her craft. Knitting was her lifelong profession. In fact, she was audited for the Guinness Book of World Records! Just like blinking, knitting was second nature to her. Her knitting was flawless. She hardly ever looked down at her needles and almost never dropped a stitch, not even in the movie theater. She had mastered both speed and accuracy. No one could match her. I could spend hours mesmerized by her nimble fingers, swiftly creating intricate patterns of delicate crocheted lace from a simple strand of yarn. How could she engage in heartfelt discussions and still produce such elegant, beautiful designs without even glancing at her needles? I, on the other hand, would need to pause and count stitches to ensure perfection. She made me the most exquisite sweaters and crochet tops, and my knitted fashion always remained on point. Not only was she punctual and detested wasting time, but she was also agile and managed her time efficiently by completing tasks swiftly and effectively.

Although Aunty Sultana taught me how to knit and embroider, I could never match her skill level. She was talented and very dedicated to her craft. She was resourceful as well. She taught numerous women to be enterprising and ran a small women's cooperative from her home. She trained them in knitting and using knitting machines. She was committed to empowering underprivileged women, enabling them to generate income for themselves. I admired her championing women's causes and making a difference in their lives. I aspired to grow up to be like her.

Everything seemed to be going very well for Aunty Sultana until the year 2000 when she was diagnosed with cancer. She had nasopharyngeal cancer, a rare form of the disease that made surgery impossible. She underwent multiple rounds of chemotherapy and radiation at AIIMS (All India Institute of Medical Sciences) in New Delhi. The illness and the treatment altered her life forever. It transformed her appearance, her voice, her eating habits, and her ability to engage in everyday activities that were once meaningful to her. She underwent a tracheostomy—a surgical incision in her throat. A thin, long tube was inserted in her throat to remove excess phlegm. She had a machine at home and, twice a day, her caregiver supported her with removing extra phlegm from her throat. If left unattended, the phlegm would cause her to choke. The removal of the phlegm brought her relief.

Her very talented daughter Amber and I share cherished memories of her.

"My mother was an incredibly positive person," says Amber. "She remained a fighter until the end. She embraced many challenges and lived her life to the fullest. Of course, she had her difficult days, but the incision in her throat and the loss of her voice became a positive part of her life because she was grateful to be alive. It didn't bother her or prevent her from doing the things she loved. She still enjoyed shopping, tending to her garden, and meeting people. She was very independent until the very end. She possessed immense strength to endure so many years in this state."

Amber remembers that her mother would visit restaurants even though she could not eat their food. "Instead, she would bring her own meal or have lunch at home before joining us. She simply relished the company of others and the lively ambiance. She loved accompanying me to my friends' homes, meeting them, traveling, and going for drives. Sometimes, during lengthy meetings, she insisted on joining me. While I attended my meetings, she would sit in the car, happily knitting away and gazing out the window. She thoroughly enjoyed those moments."

Aunty Sultana was a fashion diva and had a penchant for dressing up;

blingy rings were her signature style! She delighted in trying on various outfits and accessories. In 2011, after triumphing over cancer, she had an absolute blast walking the ramp at Pinktober, a fundraising fashion show presented by Imperial Hotel and Cancer Patients Aid Association in collaboration with fashion designer Satya Paul. It was held at the Imperial Hotel in New Delhi. She transformed her own struggle into an opportunity to make a difference for those dealing with cancer. She never slowed down, never ceased to show up for the people she loved and cared for, and never stopped pursuing her passion.

When she learned about my cancer diagnosis, she was devastated. I was in Canada at the time, and she was restless with worry. I have no doubt that she would have been there for me if she could. Despite the distance, she comforted me with her love and prayers during our phone calls.

The sound of her raspy throat lingers in my ears from our last conversation: "When will you come to India?" She struggled to hear clearly, and I struggled to understand every word she whispered on the phone. But none of that diminished the overwhelming rush of love I felt in my heart when I spoke with her. Our connection ran deep in our blood, even though we were separated by miles.

She was love. She was an inspiration. She was contribution. She was my dear Aunty Sultana.

She lives on.

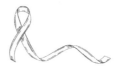

CHAPTER ONE

CANCER WAS THE CURE

by Shirin Ariff

The sun played tricks on that chilly winter day in 2013. I remember it as if it happened just yesterday. I made my way toward St. Joseph's Hospital, a mere block away from my home. A sense of anxiety consumed me. *Why did I need to see an oncologist?* I knew all too well what that word implied. This was my first appointment with an oncologist, and I hoped that Dr. Harmantas would finally provide the answers I had been desperately seeking. After months of feeling that something was amiss, I sensed that this visit might bring clarity to my questions. Even though my family doctor had dismissed my concerns about the lump on my clavicle, I *knew* deep down that something was not right. My body could *feel* it.

Terrifying thoughts filled my mind as I imagined the fate of my kids if I were to succumb to this disease. I couldn't help but wonder if I had brought this upon myself. For a long time, I had secretly harbored selfish desires for death without considering the impact on my kids. I had wished for it repeatedly, as it seemed like the only way to escape the constant and excruciating inner pain I felt each day. I longed for release from the never-ending struggle, convinced that my life held no significance and I was destined for failure.

The Breakdown

While contemplating my own mortality, I was also facing the realization that my second marriage was crumbling. I had failed miserably to earn

1

the love and loyalty of my husband. I questioned whether I was truly adequate for him. I felt humiliated, rejected, emotionally deprived, and wronged for being a trusting partner. I was hurt and deeply unhappy.

Simple, everyday tasks became Herculean tasks for me. Every morning, I had to drag myself out of bed and force myself through the day. But I felt an obligation to show up for my children. As a devoted mother, I had to put on a facade of normalcy so that my four young children could have an emotionally stable home to grow up in. I wanted that for them, and I did my best to maintain it. However, internally, I was unraveling. It was a constant battle to keep my fragmented pieces together so that I could continue to be there for my children as a complete human being.

My physical health deteriorated, serving as a clear manifestation of my inner turmoil. The winter months of 2012 were particularly challenging. I experienced multiple bouts of flu, and a small lump appeared on my left clavicle. I would often run my hands over the bump, gently pressing it to check for any pain. The lump itself did not bother me much, but I did notice that I became easily breathless and occasionally felt light-headed. My family doctor assured me that the swollen lymph node was merely doing its job of fighting off germs, possibly a lingering effect of the prolonged flu. He advised me that it would subside in a few weeks. Yet, a couple of months later, as spring approached, the lump persisted. When I revisited the doctor, he maintained his belief that it was nothing to worry about.

Then, one day, I experienced a more severe episode. I felt light-headed and struggled to breathe. Panic took hold, and I immediately called 911. The paramedics arrived at my home, causing great distress to my children, and transported me to St. Joe's in an ambulance.

After a thorough examination in the emergency room, the doctors concluded that everything was fine. I returned home a few hours later, bewildered by what was happening to me.

Despite all tests indicating otherwise, something within me still felt off. I knew deep down that something was wrong. So, I insisted that my family doctor provide a requisition for an ultrasound. It was a good thing that I did so because the ultrasound is what eventually led to concerns that there may be the possibility of cancer.

Over the course of five months, I underwent more tests and scans.

Meanwhile, amidst my own health battles, I was also navigating the process of legally separating from my husband, which only amplified my fears about the future of my children. My soon-to-be ex-husband vowed to prolong the divorce settlement until my demise. At that moment, all that mattered to me were my children. Sarah was nineteen, my twins were six, and little Simrah was three.

When the test results finally came in, it was official. I had metastatic papillary thyroid cancer. Metastatic because it had spread to my lymph nodes. And so, I found myself in a patient room, awaiting my turn to meet Dr. Harmantas.

As the doctor entered the room and took a seat in front of me, his presence was peaceful. His clean-shaven head radiated an aura that seemed to form a halo around him. He appeared as serene as Buddha. His eyes were so peaceful and meditative. In his presence, I felt a profound healing energy. He was a beacon of light.

That moment is etched in my memory forever. Leaning forward, he spoke in the softest voice, "It is cancer." Only *he* could have delivered such dreadful news with such kindness, cushioning the blow with his gentle demeanor. "You will be fine. We will take care of you," he assured me. The way he spoke those words filled me with hope. I had already placed my trust in him.

A team of doctors was assembled to support me. They had assured me that this kind of cancer could be managed. However, the reports said that the cancer cells were aggressive. They were tall cell variants (TCV), which meant we would need to intensify our efforts to treat the disease. I was in stage III, possibly even stage IV, and surgery was necessary.

The night before the surgery was the most difficult for me and for my children. It proved to be far more challenging than facing my own mortality because now I saw the situation through the eyes of my children. They were heartbroken and scared.

I was their only parent, the one who showed up for them in every aspect of their lives. I never missed a concert, a school event, any birthdays, or playdates.

My parents and siblings in India were equally stressed and worried, especially my father. It tormented him to be unable to be by my side during the most challenging period of my life. He had always been there for me. It was how we dealt with my breakdowns. He knew that I needed his comforting presence during those moments. He was my therapy, my nurturing and loving anchor—the secret sauce behind my biggest comebacks. He was my rock.

While I battled endless "what-ifs," my daughter Sarah's own world was crumbling. She worked nights at a fast food restaurant and studied Psychology at York University during the day. Her job at the restaurant funded her undergraduate studies.

Upon receiving my diagnosis, Sarah found it impossible to focus on anything. She could no longer perform her duties effectively and was forced to quit. Consumed by the fear of what the future held, she imagined a world without me and being left to care for her three siblings. Having just turned nineteen, she wasn't prepared to take on the role of a substitute mother.

In parallel to my experiences, Sarah faced her own share of hardships. As a mother, I tried to imagine what she was feeling: What was it like for her to be in a new country? What was it like for her to attend a new school? What was it like for her to have a stepfather who had committed to be there for her but had no time or love to offer her after she landed in Canada? He felt entitled to make her and me feel obligated to him for the huge favor he had done to us and demanded her obedience while showing no interest in nurturing her as a father would.

Before she arrived here with me, Sarah was loved and nurtured by my father. However, here, she felt alone. I was no longer available to sit with her every day, playing computer games and giggling over silly things. We missed our precious "Sarah and Mommy" times. Leisure time became a luxury, filed away under fond memories, like those we had in India. My life had become too busy. I had chores to do and had to manage my ex-husband's businesses, which only grew busier as his business expanded and our family grew. Sarah ceased being the baby of the house; she had to step into the role of big sister for her twin siblings. It was expected that she would babysit while I worked. We had no other help. I had to fulfill my various responsibilities as a wife, mother, secretary, office administrator, interpreter, property manager, and cleaner. It felt as if I had been brought to Canada for free labor.

November 27, 2013, marked the day of my surgery. I walked to the hospital alone, uncertain if I would ever return. The fear of mortality pounded my heart. I informed the mediators about the desired outcome for my divorce settlement and explained the need to pause the proceedings due to my serious health condition. In the operating room, as the anesthesia was administered, I experienced something completely new and unexpected. The anxiety dissipated, replaced by a pivotal moment of total surrender. Suddenly, I found myself accepting everything life had thrown at me. I took responsibility for allowing so much to happen. I wish I had better words to describe it, but all I can say is that it was the most powerful moment of my life.

Instead of fear and anxiety, my four beautiful children and my father occupied my thoughts as I slipped away under the anesthesia. I remember pleading with God for one chance to live. Childhood dreams unfolded before me like a movie. As a young girl, I had always been a dreamer, spending countless nights stargazing and envisioning who I would become when I grew up. My life and how I had lived thus far played out before my eyes.

And in that moment, I chose life—my life. Cancer, it turns out, was the *cure*. It took cancer to jolt me out of my stupor. Cancer was a gift of life. It *granted* me life, saving me from feeling dead and disconnected from myself. It rescued me from living a life I did not desire and from dying a little bit every day. It ignited an insatiable hunger to live my vision, and I began to savor life again, just like I had as a child.

According to the doctor's report, the risks of the surgery included "recurrent nerve injury with associated voice change, permanent hypo-glycemia, spinal accessory nerve injury, and shoulder weakness."

The risks were high, but the reward would be a second chance at life.

My surgery was successful, with very few side effects except for a voice change. I did not suffer any nerve injury.

Following the surgery, the oncology surgeon's report on my metastatic papillary thyroid cancer detailed the procedure: a total thyroidectomy and a bilateral central neck dissection. Yes, my neck incision ran from below my left ear to the middle of my neck, right above my right collarbone. It also involved the re-implantation of the left inferior parathyroid gland. No one knew if the parathyroid gland would function again after reimplantation, but the doctors did their best.

In his report, Dr. Harmantas also mentioned a "rock-hard" mass in the middle of the thyroid gland, almost as hard as a tennis ball. The report stated, "The jugular vein draped over the top of the tumor."

It was also noted that there were very bulky lymph nodes resembling a cluster of grapes. The report indicated that the vagus nerve and carotid artery were not involved in the disease. *Truly, miracles and the power of prayers!* I am immensely grateful to the Big G above for the gift of a second chance at life.

The surgery notes continued: "… the patient tolerated the procedure well. She returned to the recovery room in satisfactory condition." My profound sense of gratitude prevents me from taking this sentence lightly. I treasure this report as a testimony to the countless miracles that occurred in my life during that crucial time.

Within a day of returning home from the surgery, I had to rush back to the hospital because my calcium level had dropped, causing tingling sensations in my hands and feet. I had to stay in the hospital until my calcium level reached a healthy range before being discharged. In March 2014, I had to go back to St. Joe's for oral chemotherapy. Dr. Arab-O'Brien, my endocrinologist, has always had my back since my surgery. She was thorough and wanted to ensure that any remnants of cancer cells were destroyed through chemotherapy. She was my warrior woman; kind and supportive. She explained the entire process to me so that I knew what to expect. I was afraid of losing my hair and damaging my teeth. While it did affect my teeth (I now have more fillings), thankfully, nothing happened to my "crowning glory," my hair. I still struggle with chewing and swallowing food due to my "dry mouth." I have to wash down the food by drinking water. On the other hand, I tend to salivate more while speaking. If only Prime Minister Trudeau knew that "speaking moistly" has been a challenge for me ever since I underwent chemotherapy!

Ingesting the nuclear medicine and keeping it down in my stomach without throwing up became my primary mission. The medicine came in the form of a "pill" that resembled a tiny ampoule from a radio circuit. The doctor who administered the nuclear medicine arrived at my room in a hazmat suit to protect himself from the radioactive energy I was about to swallow. No one was permitted to enter my room, and I could have no visitors. The nurses left my food outside my door on a small table designated for that purpose. The doctor was the only person allowed to enter my room, clad in protective gear. All furniture and the telephone were wrapped in plastic. My movement within the room was restricted, and I was asked not to touch anything unnecessarily as I was literally radioactive. Taped paths on the floor guided me from the bed to the toilet and bathtub, and I was instructed to walk only on the tape. All faucets and flushes were covered. I had brought my towel and toiletries with me, just in case, and I was advised to keep them.

This was an unusual moment in my life. It was the first time I wouldn't see my children in person until the doctor deemed me ready to go home. I was completely alone. Sarah gave me a book, *Dying to Be Me*, by Anita

Moorjani, and I had a *tasbih* (prayer beads) to pray with. I spent a lot of time waiting by the window, gazing at Lake Ontario while reflecting, praying, or reading Anita's book. I contemplated my children, my father, and my family back home, especially those who had experienced cancer. I began to take stock of my life. My most significant takeaway from the book was the realization that when we transition, we leave everything behind. Relationships, possessions, achievements, titles, physical bodies, and even our names are relinquished in death. The only thing we carry over is the love we receive from others. Love is the currency that holds value on the other side. We carry with us the love we gave during our time on Earth and the love we received in return. This profound insight, derived from Anita's firsthand experience, has remained with me. It is why I am committed to leaving this world with an abundance of love.

My illness forced Sarah to take on many of my responsibilities. I owe a significant part of my recovery to her. Cancer provided absolute clarity about who my true family was. She became a surrogate mother to her siblings. Meanwhile, my separated husband chose to go on vacation to Chicago during my time of struggle, leaving our children to face this predicament alone as a family. It clarified for me what his commitments were and where his heart truly lay.

Sometimes, I wonder how Sarah would have managed everything on her own if it weren't for the love and support of a few parents at my children's school. Teni and Sarb took the lead. Teni was my best friend, and our children were best friends in school. Sarb, on the other hand, was a well-known figure in the neighborhood. She had twins, just like me, and our twins attended the same school, sometimes were even in the same class. Sarb was the heart of our Roncy neighborhood, and she remains so to this day.

I leaned on Teni for emotional support. She was aware of what was happening in my life and showed great kindness to me and my children. Teni organized a roster for moms who would cook and send food to my children while I was away for my surgery and chemotherapy. They took turns cooking for us and hosting my younger children for sleepovers, giving Sarah some much-needed rest. The following day, they would drop off my kids at school. These mom friends have been my angels, making this world a beautiful place. As long as we have people like them, there is hope for humanity.

The teachers at school empowered my children with love and support, along with occasional snacks. Some days, teachers would spend their lunchtime eating with my children and playing chess with them, offering extra time and attention. My parents, siblings, and new sister-in-law (my brother's wife) offered countless prayers from India for my miraculous recovery.

My school friends organized global prayer chains, and whenever they traveled, they remembered me and offered special prayers. Prayers were said worldwide in mosques, temples, and churches. My childhood friend Nancy even prayed at the statue of Madonna, standing in the freezing cold winter snow before dawn, to ask God to heal me. Love and prayers surrounded me; I am blessed and grateful for each and every one of them. On the other hand, none of my in-laws bothered to inquire about us, not even those who would reach out to me solely for their own interests. They turned their backs on us.

But I had found my real family.

The greatest lesson I learned was to stay true to myself and live my life authentically. That was the legacy I wanted to leave for my children. Before cancer, I hadn't been living a life of my own choice. I was living by default, believing I had no other option. As a woman, it was expected of me to make all the adjustments and compromises in life. I was supposed to prioritize everyone else in my family and always put them before myself. That was the mark of a good woman. For a long time, I conformed to the rules and expectations imposed on me by others. From education to marriage and motherhood, the expectations were clear:

I had to complete my formal education by my early twenties.

I should be married and become a mother by my mid-twenties.

After my first marriage ended, I *had to* remarry again in my early thirties because I was too young to live my life alone.

I *had to* have all my children before my forties.

And there was this: If I didn't adhere to my husband's rules, I would be deported, and my children would be taken away from me.

The list went on.

The *should-haves* and *must-dos* had a firm grip on my life, and the real risk of losing everything loomed over me if I failed to comply. The pressure to conform to the predetermined path set by family and society was overwhelmingly heavy.

I had been living my life according to deadlines and ultimatums imposed by others. I was a prisoner of my own beliefs, enslaved by the need to please everyone else, even though I remained desperately unhappy. I had lost all appreciation for my own life. It had become burdensome, weighed down by repressed anger, and I placed blame on others for everything that went wrong. Until I experienced cancer.

Breaking Through

Cancer became the most profound and powerful lesson in my life, teaching me what no amount of formal education or degrees ever could. It cracked me open. It became a catalyst for accessing my personal power and cultivating a culture of self-love and self-trust. I chose to learn this lesson at the cost of almost losing my life. Experiencing cancer awakened my love for myself, instilling a deep gratitude for life and the people I encountered along the way. It became an intensive course in various life lessons.

According to Darryl D'Souza, a healer from India, I had "tremendous emotional agony and trauma trapped at a cellular level." My sister, who is also a healer in India, shared numerous spiritual and healing modalities with me. This marked the beginning of my spiritual journey as I sought healing and transformation from within. I delved into mindfulness, spirituality, emotional intelligence, and personal development through various courses. The more I explored myself on this journey of self-mastery, the more I hungered for knowledge and growth. It was a comforting, soothing, therapeutic, empowering, and liberating process. Powerful healers emerged to assist me on my path. I relished being in a space of complete self-acceptance and surrender, discovering a world of compassionate and selfless individuals who supported me without any hidden agendas. I let go of inherited belief patterns and embraced whatever brought me peace. I shattered the barriers of organized religion, perceiving them as different expressions of the same concepts. I expanded within the openness of my spiritual experiences, capable of visiting places of worship and religious sanctuaries without being constrained by limiting beliefs.

My most significant breakthroughs came when I attended personal development and leadership programs that taught me to release blame, shame, complaints, and resentment. The shift occurred when I chose to forgive not only others but also myself for the choices I made. Forgiveness was not instantaneous; it was a gradual process of growth and transformation that I experienced. It was the most challenging, ongoing, and profound experience that caused my heart to burst open.

I discovered that we don't see things as *they are*; we see them as *we are*. I encountered a whole new version of myself as a being of love, unbounded and awakened to the understanding that there was no wrongdoing and nothing to forgive. When I embraced full responsibility for everything that happened in my life, I set myself free. I freed myself from the stories I had constructed in my mind and released the grip of my past, ready to design my future on a clean slate. Armed with a powerful context for living, I rediscovered myself as a possibility of love, empowerment, and transformation, becoming a living testament to self-empowerment. As I continued this journey, the world around me became more magical. A future filled with joy and wonder unfolded before my eyes.

Although I still face moments of breakdown and occasionally battle negativity, I have acquired skills and tools to confront them powerfully. I seek guidance and support from loving and nurturing individuals.

Healing

Healing is an integral part of my life. Even to this day, I engage in meditation, which sustains and empowers me. It serves as a reset button, allowing me to live in a meditative state even while performing daily tasks such as cooking, writing, or doing chores around the house. I immerse myself fully and completely.

One of the secrets to my growth and expansion is living a life of humility. Each day, I consciously make an effort to trust the process and surrender to it. I let go of any sense of entitlement and create my world from nothingness. Some days are easier than others, and I am intentional about quickly snapping out of the quagmire of negative thoughts. I have no attachments to the results I have created in life, and I am joyful for them. In my experience, humility means recognizing my power without taking it for granted. It allows me to be a perpetual learner and creates space for continued growth. Humility does not limit my expansion; it is the key to ongoing self-mastery. It involves sacred acknowledgment and acceptance of the collaboration with a higher power—All That Is.

Knowledge flows to me as long as I remain receptive. Teachers appear when I express a willingness to learn. I continue to work on softening my being, and in doing so, healing occurs. By confronting my fears of judgment and choosing vulnerability and openness, I experience deeper healing. I remain a work in progress, and I am committed to this lifelong process. During moments of regression, my chosen family supports me, and together, we reset.

Transformation

In my meditation, I express gratitude to my cancer cells. Cancer became my cure. It performed the arduous task of healing my spirit. As the scars on my throat slowly faded away, my health was restored.

Years later, I found myself dining with my children. at an Asian restaurant. A Buddhist monk approached me. He remarked that he could see the light within me and was curious about the source of that light. I felt humbled and grateful. It inspired me to continue my personal growth. I chose not to fade into oblivion without making my life and experiences count. I dedicated my lonely nights to self-discovery and meditation. I immersed myself in powerful communities. I persevered in being a positive force in the world around me. My life is an ongoing transformation.

As a mother of three daughters and a son, I am fully present in my responsibilities as a parent. I stand in support of my daughters, encouraging them to find their voices and recognizing the power and grace within them as women. My son has been raised without any expectation of privilege solely based on his gender. He is taught not to use his gender as a means to assert power over other women. Love and respect are given and received equally among us. Being a man or woman does not alter the way we love and respect one another.

For a phase of my life, I endured immense hardship and suffering due to being a woman, grappling with emotional dependency and longing for love from those who didn't deserve me or reciprocate that love. I now forgive myself for subjecting myself to such suffering and leading a difficult life, recognizing that I didn't have to make it so arduous. I am an educated woman. I attended schools that aimed to empower women.

So, why did I compromise? I would stand up for anyone else enduring even a fraction of the suffering I experienced. What prevented me from standing up for myself? It was my desperate need to feel loved that led me to inflict harm upon myself. I had been striving relentlessly for external validation and recognition from my ex-husband and his family. My desperation for love and acceptance drove me to engage in actions that contradicted my true self. I nearly destroyed myself in the pursuit of love. What didn't work was my fixed idea of what love should look like and my limited perspective on who could provide that love. I failed to remain open to other possibilities.

Until cancer.

Cancer taught me to become the love I had been seeking in this world. Above all else, cancer taught me to love and trust myself because, in doing so, I opened myself up to experiencing the greatest love of all and tapping into my own personal power. I became my own North Star.

It's never too late
When life begins –
When you don't give up
You let courage win
—Shirin Ariff, from the poem "Now"
from Keepsake A Souvenir of Love

SHIRIN ARIFF

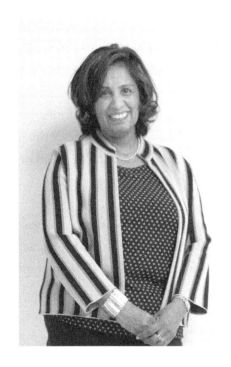

Shirin Ariff, BA (Eng. Hons.), BEd, is a five-time bestselling author and has over three million global views of her viral speech "Love Conquers All".

As a Life Transformation Coach, she equips her clients with tools and distinctions to access their own personal power and live a life of authenticity, joy, freedom, and dignity.

Shirin's own heart-wrenching story of dramatic ups and downs and her remarkable journey of resilience as a mother of four children is etched in her international bestselling book, *The Second Wife*. Shirin struggled with facial paralysis, survived cancer, and endured two failed marriages. Shirin has been there and done that. She uses her life experiences to empower others and is lovingly called "Coach Yoda."

Shirin's life story, "Beauty and the Beast," from the Dream Big docuseries by Ethnic Channel Group, was featured at the New York International Women's Film Festival and short-listed at the Toronto International Women's Film Festival 2021.

Shirin is the founding member and president of the Brampton chapter for Immigrant Women in Business, an organization dedicated to helping immigrant women succeed. Shirin represents Indo-Canadian women. Shirin serves her community as the founder of 7 Arcs Creative Works by creating inspiring books and anthologies and empowering others with her raw and unrehearsed talk show, the "Share Your Shine" series on her Be Your Own North Star YouTube channel. Shirin has hand-crafted and delivered several workshops and individual and group coaching programs under her Be Your Own North Star brand, imparting transformative learning. Shirin is also an Executive Contributor to the European-based *Brainz Magazine*, which globally features articles and stories based on leadership and mindset.

Shirin is the proud recipient of the International Women Achievers Award, 2020 as a Woman of Purpose, and the Spiritual Writer/Composer Halo Award, 2020. Shirin was nominated for the Top 25 Immigrant Women in Canada, 2022, and received the Woman on Fire Award, 2023.

Visit Shirin online at *shirinariff.com*

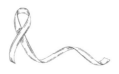

CHAPTER TWO

TOUCHED BY THE C-FAIRY

by Pat Labez

L ooking up at the iconic ball, hearing the chant of thousands of people calling out the countdown in unison: "10-9-8-7-6-5-4-3-2-1 … HAPPY NEW YEAR!!!!" Cheers, music, sounds of celebration, and confetti filled the air and decorated the streets around Times Square. Everyone hugged each other, kisses flew, and smiles and laughter were exchanged among strangers as we stood in front of Bubba Gump Shrimp restaurant, welcoming in 2013!!

And there was Joy, taking it all in—the magic of the holidays—with a look of promise and hope. I snapped a photo of her, capturing that expression of pure wonder, peace, calm, satisfaction, and resolve.

Another item checked off her bucket list.

It is said that about a million people gather annually around Times Square in New York City to ring in the New Year. I used to be one of those people who watched the festivities on television and always said, "You'd *never* see me there with all those people. That's crazy!"

But after that experience, I knew I would never say "never" again. No words can express the sheer joy of that moment, forever etched in my heart and mind.

You see, just three weeks earlier, as I prepared to have lunch with my daughter, Amanda Joy, finally feeling somewhat settled after our big move from Camarillo, California, to Austin, Texas, I received a call from my sister, Joy.

"Are you sitting down?" she asked.

"Yes," I replied, bracing myself, as she had mentioned not having much of an appetite during a recent Thanksgiving gathering with her friends. Even though she had been packed for another work assignment overseas, Joy found herself at the hospital in Washington, D.C., awaiting test results following excruciating abdominal pain.

"I guess I've been touched by the C-Fairy!" exclaimed Joy.

"What?" I asked, baffled by her choice of words.

"Yup, they say it's cancer. Three months. Can you come?"

Silence.

I choked, trying to find the "right" words to comfort, support, and simply put on that warrior suit.

Is this really what I think it is?

Questions began racing through my mind, but I didn't want to ask for fear of the answers that I would get. The events of the next few weeks are somewhat blurry. When you receive news like this, your mind can't help but go straight to "the inevitable"—the end. I found myself thinking of our brother, Nestor, who died of brain cancer at the age of eighteen on Mother's Day. Forty years later, we were facing stage IV pancreatic cancer, "the silent killer," and stage II breast cancer, "a rare and aggressive form not related to the other," as described by the doctor.

A mad scramble ensued to put parental support in place for my then-fourteen-year-old daughter, Amanda Joy. Within forty-eight hours, I was by my sister's side in Washington, meeting with doctors, nurses, interns, and a seemingly revolving door of medical staff.

"Get your affairs in order," we were told. "We're looking at one to three months."

The gravity of the situation was, of course, somewhat tempered by the magic of Christmas. And leave it to Joy, who somehow always found the goodness in all things, no matter what, to be sitting upright on her bed with a big smile on her face when I walked into her hospital room.

There she was, holding a blue balloon that said, "It's a boy!"

Let me explain: You see, for months, she had been complaining of not feeling well, of having stomach discomfort, and of not having much of an appetite. She led a busy life, but I kept encouraging her to please get checked. A prescription for acid reflux seemed to help temporarily. But the mysterious symptoms returned. So, here she was, "solving" the mystery for friends who surrounded her. Strangers who didn't know her would, of course, pass her by and say "Congratulations!" not realizing that, at fifty-eight, she was a career woman, never married, no kids, and simply happy to be Auntie Joy to many.

Joy exclaimed, "Well, I guess we're gonna have to figure out how to stop the buzzing of this *C-Fairy!*"

That urgent request marked the beginning of my own life lesson in facing your own mortality—confronting the fight of your life. It made me realize just how critical our mindset is to our overall health and wellness. Having worked in health and human services for years, I was the go-to person in the family for crisis intervention. Joy often chided me about it, saying that I'd better get used to the fact that I'd probably end up taking care of everyone. I was the youngest of nine siblings.

I thought I was up for the task.

I quickly realized that managing caregivers for others and ensuring regulatory compliance is one thing, but being the actual caregiver of a loved one was something entirely different. The physical toll would eventually catch up with me. And the emotional and mental stamina required was a whole other challenge unto itself. As if that wasn't enough, I was also charged with the responsibility of taking care of my own family calamities, including a husband scheduled for major back surgery and a teen daughter in need of ongoing physical therapy for a ballet injury.

"Keep looking up!" became our theme.

Trips to the infusion center were referred to as "going to the spa." It seemed a bit bizarre to others that we'd be packing up for the day with smiles on our faces despite the dreaded after-effects. Chemotherapy sessions became "having a cocktail."

As a matter of fact, during one of her telework conferences, apparently, a co-worker questioned why Joy was proudly talking about going to the spa and having a cocktail. *Aha! That's another lesson.* Let's not assume we know what others are really going through or be quick to judge.

Bottom line: We never gave up!

Given the hustle and bustle of the holidays (it was December 2012), the gavel came down with the news at the same time hospitals and businesses were scaling back schedules. We knew that time was of the essence. A hospital in Washington, DC (which shall remain nameless as it is not my intent to spread the word of how bad they were) had scheduled her for a January 4th infusion, the first available date after the holidays. The doctor emphasized how critical it was for her to start chemo as soon as possible. That gave them over three weeks to get the necessary insurance approvals, by the way, and prepare for this "urgent" procedure.

Rather than waiting around, where every day was another day lost, we decided to be proactive. Even though we were told that the cancer was inoperable, we set out to get second, third, and fourth opinions if needed.

We searched for the top cancer centers in the region. I was frantically faxing medical records for immediate review to see who could take Joy on as a patient. Getting timely replies was challenging, and we were running out of patience, that's for sure!

MD Anderson Cancer Center in Houston, Texas, was one option, but I firmly believe that part of the healing process is to be surrounded by your loved ones and your network, and since we didn't know a single soul in the Houston area, that option was out.

Memorial Sloan Kettering in New York? Perhaps a little better because at least my family would be there part-time. Georgetown University Hospital? The location was great, about two miles from Joy's home. Johns Hopkins Medical Center in Maryland? Great reputation, but it would entail a two-hour drive one way. Tough decisions. But at this point, it was about who could get her in ASAP while we waited for the DC hospital to take action.

After looking through websites, my sister wished for Dr. Daniel Laherul of Johns Hopkins. We knew there was no way of requesting him. But lo and behold, as we went to Baltimore for that team assessment to determine whether they'd be able to take her in, who ended up being assigned to her? Yes, Dr. Daniel Laheru!

Coincidence?

The next four years under Dr. Laheru's care would prove to be not only the most rewarding but also the roller-coaster ride of our lifetime.

Because of the urgency, we went ahead and proceeded with what we thought was already in place at the DC hospital—chemotherapy. The day before Joy was supposed to start her first treatment, I got a call. They needed to postpone treatment because they hadn't received insurance approval. They'd had more than three weeks to process the paperwork and still no insurance approval. It was deflating. We felt very anxious, especially when the oncologist had insisted that treatment was needed "yesterday."

Well, so be it. We lost five more days.

Next scheduled visit: Everything seemed to go just fine, and we were about to give a sigh of relief until, just as the nurse was about to administer the chemo, we heard, "Stop! Stop! Don't!"

What? Yup, no insurance approval! *Again.*

That was it.

Yes, there were a series of unpleasant, questionable processes we had to go through earlier, but these two incidents were enough to stop us dead cold in our tracks. Fortunately, we had already mobilized Johns Hopkins, Plan B, while waiting, and we were able to move forward with Joy's treatment there.

The Willie Nelson song "On the Road Again" became our theme song during our trips to "the spa." Yup, that song always got us started with smiles and giggles.

At some point, we'd usually change the car music to Hawaiian songs, bringing her back to the days of our youth in Hawaii. She was, after all, also a beautiful Hawaiian *hula* dancer.

We had to consider logistics. At a minimum, we needed to allow two hours' drive time from Arlington, Virginia, to Baltimore, Maryland. Together with her closest friends, we agreed that we'd simply make it happen.

We made a pact to do "Whatever it takes!"

I was comforted by the fact that if I was unable to take her in, she had an amazing network of friends who would gladly step in.

And so the journey began.

We agreed to do the recommended traditional treatment of chemotherapy and radiation. At that time, well-intended friends were bombarding us with homeopathic remedies. It was overwhelming. Somehow, we gravitated to one alternative treatment that seemed unique. As woo-woo as that may have seemed to many, we figured, "Why not?" Medical professionals and scientists assured us of its safety record, and that was enough for us.

When your life is already at stake, what else have you got to lose, right?

Yes, almost immediately, Joy responded to her treatments! There was even a fifteen-month stretch of relative calm. Ringing that bell at the radiation department to signify her last session was a huge moment.

It was then that I confessed to her doctors that I had been giving her a special supplement in addition to her hospital treatments: "It may be coincidental, but may I continue this?"

The doctor said, "Whatever you're doing, keep doing it because she's our miracle girl."

Our trips to the spa truly became an outing of sorts. Joy made friends at the infusion center as she'd bring her snacks, prayer book, notes, and inspirational material … things that brought her comfort.

We entered a new phase of the journey: Joy's pancreatic cancer seemed to have calmed down against all odds. Doctors now recommended addressing her breast cancer with a mastectomy, saying it was the only way to ensure it would not get worse. So, we started 2014 by doing exactly that.

We were flabbergasted to think that a body part is cut off and you're sent home on the same day.

"Noooooo!" I begged the hospital to keep her at least overnight. I felt inept and ill-equipped to be doing wound care. But I had to suck it up and just handle it.

Post-mastectomy care was one of the hardest things I've had to do in terms of learning how to do wound care, administer medications, and assist in all facets of activities of daily living—bathing, dressing, ambulating, etc.

In hindsight, I wish I had asked for help then. It was intense.

After Joy's thirty-day post-op checkup, we were rewarded with a resounding: "You're doing good!"

But that sigh of relief was short-lived. A few days later, I opened my eyes and—BOOM! This time, it was ME!

I couldn't move. The pain was so intense. I didn't know what was happening. *What's going on? Am I having a nightmare?*

I struggled to get out of bed but finally found my way through the fog and got myself to a physician's office.

The doctor gave me shocking news: six degenerative discs on my neck and a pea-sized brain tumor on my right temple.

"Meningioma is benign in seventy percent of cases, but we highly recommend surgery," she said, reminding us of our family history. "Even if benign, it will keep growing and should be removed."

We moved on as best we could. I did my regular, quarterly MRIs, knowing the best case I could hope for was keeping the tumor from growing. Doctors insisted I really needed to have surgery in anticipation of the tumor's continued growth, which would put pressure on my brain.

I opted to wait and told them, "I'll take my chances."

I was taking a leap of faith.

"I'm not afraid of dying. When it's my time, it's my time."

I was hopeful that "the pea" could somehow just behave and leave me alone, at least long enough for me to help those relying on me.

The insanity of life continued with the day-to-day struggles of survival.

Every time I'd get a headache, I wondered if that was the pea acting up. Somehow, I managed to function. I conducted even more research on cellular health and the supplement that I was giving Joy, then opted to get on it, feeling that it was my only chance to avoid prescriptions and their side effects.

Focusing on others was really my chosen therapy, along with lifestyle adjustments, gratitude, and prayer. I figured Joy was already beating the odds and wondered if any of that had made a difference.

In many ways, I believe my focus on taking care of others really meant having no time to worry about myself—between my young daughter's injuries and pain management struggles through her teen years, my husband's pending back surgery, and my sister's fight for her life. I think it was all about survival at that point. It was about learning not to take anything for granted and enjoying every day we are given, no matter what challenges we face. Things could be better, but things could always be worse.

I tried to find humor in every day-to-day situation.

And the beat went on.

Joy amazingly kept on working, albeit mostly remotely. There were many times when she'd be on a conference call as I gently massaged her back with her favorite therapeutic gel. Everyone questioned why she didn't just retire. Her answer was that she didn't want to spend her days focusing on her situation. Work gave her purpose and allowed her to focus on something other than herself.

Her most recent assignment had something to do with overseeing U.S. support and funding of various food programs in Africa. Her job took her to remote villages in Third World countries, keeping her grounded in the goodness of our country and the freedom and opportunities available that others can only wish for.

Fast forward to 2016. We both kept each other afloat emotionally and mentally. The fact that four years had passed and she was hanging on was a gift we truly embraced. Likewise, the fact that my MRIs turned from quarterly to bi-annual was a good sign. Additionally, it was Amanda Joy's high school graduation and the year she turned eighteen. Joy had milestones that kept her going.

"Take Amanda Joy to Europe, Pat. It'll open up her world."

And so, I set out to do just that. At the same time, I was also preparing to be an empty nester, recognizing that a new chapter was unfolding in my life.

Things seemed to be under control.

In anticipation of Amanda's graduation, I returned to volunteering, along with my health advocacy initiatives. It's a good way to serve, expand my purpose, and meet new people.

After years in long-term care, I needed a change from the emotional drain of caregiving and loss, so I opted for something more creative, going back to my earlier roots as a performer. I chose a film lab to escape the "big unknown" of my future. I was asked for a talent directory headshot. I resisted but ultimately agreed. Why not? A week later, I received an invitation to audition for a short film. *Well, surprise, surprise!* After twenty-five years of having walked away from show business, this was definitely unexpected!

Intrigued by the whole thing, I said, "Why not?"

While Joy made it to New York City for Amanda's graduation, she opted to stay behind for our European escapade and just asked for photographs throughout the adventure. One day, I checked in on her from Edinburgh Castle in Scotland, and her voice was faint.

She whispered, "I'm not well." It was Independence Day.

I flew right back and found her on the couch, curled up in the dark. We hugged, sat side by side, and held each other.

No words. Just being together, sensing each other's thoughts.

It was the roughest part of the journey, witnessing firsthand the pain and agony of the body succumbing to disease while the spirit fought on through Christmas and into the New Year.

No matter what, she managed to smile, joke, and bring joy to anyone around her. In solitude, she loved her Hawaiian and gospel music playing in the background.

Then I got the call—an offer in a short film. The role: a mom dying of cancer. Coincidence? I was about to turn it down. I was uncomfortable leaving Joy for the three-day filming in New York, but she said, "Why not, Pat? What is there to think about? You need to do this. You've given this up for far too long. *Follow your destiny.* You must do this. Go, I'll be fine." I accepted the role.

* * *

Joy convinced me to *embrace life* and do it, even with my own brain tumor … or perhaps even more *because* of my brain tumor—a reminder of how fragile life is.

On January 22, 2017, as our favorite Hawaiian song played, "Kanaka Wai Wai" ("Let Me Walk Through Paradise with You, Lord"), her beautiful, tender *hula* hands lay lifeless.

"Take my hand and lead me there," floated across the room as Joy took her last breath.

Coincidence?

With friends and family by her side, love and light permeated the room.

I felt numb but kept quiet, focusing on the tasks at hand. Perhaps it was denial, fear, or disbelief, but we were convinced she could beat this to the end, right up until the moment she was placed in a body bag. Down the elevator. Loaded up in the trunk of a station wagon. That was it.

Five days later, I was asked to identify her. Clinging on to each other, my friend Joann and I walked into the mortuary, not quite knowing what to expect. A few yards away, we could see a body in a plain gray cardboard casket at the front of the room. For a moment, we stayed back, unsure if we were intruding on someone else's I.D. viewing. The funeral aide nodded.

"That's her?" I asked.

Joann and I just looked at each other, quietly dumbfounded. Ever so slowly, we walked up. Other than her pink top, nothing else seemed recognizable.

I looked her over, shaking, confused, and shocked, asking myself, "This is Joy?"

Looking hard, I guess I could see some resemblance between the family features. But she seemed empty, like a somewhat deflated balloon.

It was then that I knew and understood.

That was not Joy.

It was merely a shell to house her beautiful spirit that's now soaring, pain-free, celebrating life again without the confines of her earthly body.

Relief and a sense of peace washed over me, easing the heaviness in my heart since her passing. As I accepted this spiritual awareness and connection, the freedom of our soul beyond this life, my perception of living changed. The *manini* ("trivial" in Hawaiian) lost their importance. What mattered was staying healthy—in spirit, body, and relationships. So, I moved on. Aware and cognizant of the importance of stress management for my own health and wellness, I went about life, taking care of whatever was necessary for final arrangements.

"Anytime you're ready," the gentleman said.

I shook, took a deep breath, and with a flick of a switch, I could hear the motor activate behind me. I turned around and saw my Joy—my beloved sister and best friend—being rolled into the chamber.

At a distance, I could see a light. It was the end of a journey. Just like that.

She was the planner in the family. She had the plots and funeral arrangements done years beforehand. But flicking that switch was never an option given before. I was conflicted, feeling like I, myself, was setting her on fire. But I decided to embrace the moment as a gift, traveling right with her from start to finish.

I drew strength from the handful of loving friends watching from behind the glass window and her *Kumu*, her *hula* teacher, right beside me.

"She's up in the big *luau*, celebrating with the others!" he said, smiling. He opened his jacket to reveal a white Hawaiian shirt made of the same material as the white *muumuu* on Joy. An unexpected video showing a tropical beach ran behind us, bringing us back to our roots in Hawaii.

Coincidence?

Joy was so loved; we had a Celebration of Life in Washington to honor her with the many friends she had made throughout her twenty-six-year residency in the area. Then, as she wished, her final Celebration of Life followed a month later in Hawaii, overlooking the panoramic Ko'olau mountain range and the Pacific Ocean, resting in the same vault as our beloved brother, Zach. To everyone, he was her "dance partner." To Joy, he was her soul mate, and she'd always say, "I miss him."

As I danced the same *hula* she taught me—to the song that was playing as she took her last breath—a beautiful white dove mysteriously flew behind me across the indoor stage.

Coincidence?

The path to healing was still a long road to walk. I had *my* life to live and attend to family needs.

To stay motivated, I adopted the mantra, "Find Joy in the Journey." It seemed to help me cope and focus on the goodness in things, people, and situations rather than the imperfections and ongoing challenges of life. The mantra renewed my appreciation of everything, especially health. I tried to imagine how Joy might have lived. *Carpe Diem!* was another sentiment I used to live by but had forgotten. I brought it back. Yes, "Seize the Day!" It was back to living in the moment with my signature "go with the flow, come what may" mindset.

Whenever another crisis came up, I'd simply say, "Bring it on!"

Through it all, I'd find humor in everything, a silver lining through every adversity.

"Is this for real?" I'd often ask.

After the passing of another friend to pancreatic cancer, I felt compelled to produce a short film, *Howard*, a love story inspired by two very special people I met through Joy. At its screening, I was asked if this was something Joy and I had discussed. It wasn't. Apparently, Joy had been wanting to share the story many years earlier. And on the day of screening, wishing she was there to witness its unveiling, I opened my computer and stumbled on her last *hula* performance at the Smithsonian National Museum of the American Indian in D.C., dancing to *He Hawaii Au*. It's as if she had returned to celebrate with us.

The film received the Audience Choice Award at the Asian Pacific American Film Festival, and a feature film is in the works.

Did Joy have a hand in this, too?

Later that year, another family loss in Hawaii took place with the passing of my brother-in-law, Harold. I spent over a month there, helping my sister, Alma. Upon my return, I realized I hadn't had my regular MRIs! With no symptoms whatsoever and sheer busyness, I'd forgotten about my little pea!

When I finally scheduled a scan, the doctor said, "Pat, check your MRI. We could not find the tumor. It's all good!"

"What?! How?! When?!" I was perplexed. But it doesn't matter. I accepted—the gift of health, the gift of life—with deep gratitude.

I've always said, "I'm not afraid to die." Yet, I now realize that perhaps "I was afraid to live" also held true. I find it ironic that I've come full circle as my journey of introspective understanding at sixty-three is what I started at twenty-three, thwarted by, and yet enriched with, life lessons.

As a young adult, I heard the phrase, "Life is not a dress rehearsal." It may have taken a lifetime, but I finally see it now.

I believe there are no coincidences and that all things happen for a reason. Embarking on your fight for life, believe that it's truly about living in the moment, as the future is promised to no one. With the flick of a switch, life changes. And the body is merely a costume for our spirit.

We're all performers on the stage of life, improvising along the way until the journey ends with your final curtain call. Make the most of it. Do good. Be good. Blessings are everywhere, often simply disguised.

Even so-called disappointments can later uncover opportunity and joy beyond imagination.

Yes, through all the ups and downs, zigzags, and detours of life, every one of us can find joy in the journey!

Why my beloved sister, Joy, might have been "Touched by the C-Fairy," I can't say for sure. I do know that those who were fortunate enough to know her were "Touched by an Angel," which happened to be the title of a favorite TV show of ours. The show served as a good reminder that angels in many forms are around us, offering many valuable life lessons if only we'd stop long enough to recognize them. But, of course, for many of us, the daily grind of making a living often takes over, and we forget that making a living is not the same as truly "living" to our fullest.

They say the First Act in life is when we learn the skills to navigate through life. The Second Act is when we focus on our career, marriage, kids, and family. The Third Act is about the pursuit of wisdom, self-actualization, and leaving some kind of a legacy.

So, I challenge you to pick one thing you've always wanted to do and do it. If physical limitations are a deterrent, how about something such as sharing your wisdom? We all have stories. Life lessons are priceless.

Years ago, when I volunteered for hospice, using a cassette tape to record stories seemed like the most precious gift I could give to their families. I can't tell you how many times folks would express such deep gratitude. "Thank you so much. I never knew that about Mom (or Dad, or another loved one)!"

Consider recording your life lessons, wisdom, and memories. It doesn't have to be a whole book's worth if that seems daunting.

Just do a chapter ... a snippet ... a special path you may have taken in the journey of life. Your words could make a lasting impact on someone else.

As long as the heart is beating, there is hope. And happiness is always on standby. The universe isn't done with us yet. Go. Live your joy. Leave that mark ... that footprint of yours.

How are you doing with your bucket list? Or have you cast that aside because life just got in the way? You might wanna check in once in a while.

Recently, a special event took me to the shores of Fort Erie, Ontario, Canada. I realized it was near Niagara Falls, and I was suddenly reminded that a visit to Niagara Falls was on Joy's bucket list. I had no idea how close it was to New York, and we promised each other that we'd treat ourselves to that "next time."

Well, "next time" never came. And so, I made the decision to put it on MY bucket list in memory of Joy.

My friend, Catherine, offered to join me and, thanks to her, I made it a point to get to Niagara Falls up close and personal, feeling and hearing the roaring power of Mother Nature in all her grandeur, yet having an amazingly calming effect at the same time. I could sense peace. And Joy. A rainbow even appeared through the mist of the Falls. It was beautiful. It was magical. It was another memory etched in my heart and mind, another acknowledgment of how we need to listen to these spiritual whispers as they come.

As the saying goes, "Life is a gift that keeps on giving," and I believe that "a joyful heart is the beat of life."

Five years after that agonizing decision to accept the role of the dying mother and miss the precious company of my dying sister for a few days, I felt more alive than ever. My biggest cheerleader was my sister, smiling away as she watched the rough cut of that film.

She never made it to the live screening in New York that spring. But, yes, I believe her spirit lives. And, thanks to her, so does mine.

My Third Act has been a series of beautiful surprises and wonders, with no signs of slowing down anytime soon. Well, the *New England Journal of Medicine* cited those folks in their 50s, 60s, 70s, and 80s are actually in the most productive stage of their life, and I am certainly a living example of that. Not only am I continuing with acting but expanding projects wherever I can be of service. I find all of it amazingly fulfilling, beyond anything I could've ever imagined.

You see, I am constantly reminded that, with a flick of a switch, life can change. Just as sudden as the discovery of that tumor was and as mysterious as its disappearance four years later, with or without the C-Fairy, I was reminded again of how fragile life is.

I started out in 2022 with a concussion when I took a fall while visiting Amanda Joy in England over the holidays. Eventually, a series of tests would lead to the discovery of another brain tumor.

Coincidence?

What the future holds is anyone's guess. But I know I will live my life to the fullest wherever I may be on this journey.

I do hope you'll do the same.

Please reach out to someone, me included, for resources, ideas, and programs that you or someone you love may be able to tap into and benefit from.

Yes, this is not a dress rehearsal. And until the curtain closes, let's give ourselves permission to perform—in whatever form that performance may be—whether it's doing, learning, or teaching something, know that you can have a life that may even surpass the First and Second Acts of life. You may even have a grand Third Act … an ENCORE! Bravo!

And while you're at it, remember to look for the sunbeams and rainbows in the waterfalls of life—you just might spot a fairy sprinkling joy and hope—a reminder to seize the day! With a flick of a switch, life can change.

PAT LABEZ

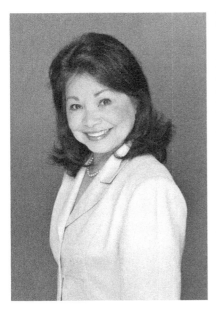

Pat Labez, often hailed as "The Joyful Sage," has devoted her life to championing seniors. An international bestselling author, accomplished actress, producer, and speaker, Pat collaborates with older adults to enhance joy and redefine retirement through the arts. With a background as a certified administrator for a residential care facility for the elderly, Pat received accolades for outstanding health-care services. Additionally, she held a prominent position as the director of human resources and volunteer services for a county-wide health and human-services agency.

Melding her professional journey with her passion for performing arts, Pat founded Third Act Encore and serves on the board of the International Mental Health Foundation. Furthermore, she leads as the Chapter President of Nexus Network International.

Launching her television career over three decades ago in Hawaii, Pat made an inspiring comeback to the entertainment world in her 60s after bravely overcoming a brain tumor. Her renewed career boasts roles in TV shows like *Blue Bloods, New Amsterdam*, and *The Other Two*. Moreover, her involvement extends to film, theater, and musicals, either as a producer or performer.

With an extensive history of volunteering, Pat has contributed to organizations like the Alzheimer's Association, AARP, RSVP, Council on Aging, Hospice, and the American Red Cross. Together with her team, Pat guides families through retirement challenges, empowering them to embrace their "Third Act"—a phase characterized by wisdom, self-fulfillment, and the pursuit of leaving a legacy.

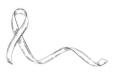

CHAPTER THREE

LOOK AT ME

by CoCo Roper

I may only be twenty-nine years old, but I have already lived many different lives. Surprisingly it is *this* life—the one infiltrated by cancer, surgeries, mobility aids, and the fight of my life—that saved me.

I come from a family that has always been in the spotlight. From the outside looking in, we were like the Costa Rican version of the Kardashians. My mother was always in the spotlight. She was Puerto Rican, drop-dead gorgeous, and a socialite. In the 90s, she was even crowned Miss Puerto Rico. Her husbands and our entire family have been featured in countless Puerto Rican and Costa Rican news and entertainment magazines throughout our lives. This is because people were dazzled by the glamor, fashion, fame, and money that surrounded us—and the drama, of course.

Despite having fans following our every move as a family, outsiders only saw about ten percent of the reality of our fractured lives.

When I was four and a half, my mother divorced my biological father. Their marriage had been volatile at the best of times. My father had demanded my mother give up a lot of what she loved, such as modeling, working on television, and building her brand to be a stay-at-home mother and ideal wife to him. Their marriage was destined to fail, and when it did, my nightmare began.

I would see my biological father for two days every other week after they split up. On these visits, we'd be a real family during the day. My sister, half-brother, dad, and I would chase each other around the expansive property on ATVs, have barbeques, swim in the pool, and even drink underage. Most of all, we would spend time together like a family, which is all any of us kids wanted.

But at night, things changed for me *and* my sister (though I didn't know it at the time). From age five, my biological father sexually abused me. And it broke me. He never touched me while he was with my mom. But once she left, it was torture. The abuse continued until I was nine and got my period—thank God I got it earlier than most other girls.

I get into it much more in my book, but for now, try to understand that my abuse marked the beginning of a lifelong inability to love myself or my body in any healthy way. It led to a lifetime of self-destruction, pain, addiction, and reinvention. It may even, in some way, have led to my cancer.

Incredibly, when I wasn't at my father's house, I lived a fairytale life. I would push down everything that happened on the weekend and live a celebrity life. My mom married Gary, who became my stepfather. And I adored him. He had more money than my mother, sister, or I had ever seen in real life. It was everywhere. We had maids, bodyguards, barred windows (for our protection), and armored vehicles. We were watched everywhere we went. There was no privacy. Every move, event, or mistake was at risk of being blown out of proportion and connected to our mother. That meant our lives demanded beauty, perfection, and high fashion. At age ten, I was wearing Burberry heels and carrying Louis Vuitton bags. By the time I was eleven or twelve years old, I was in bars, wearing skin-tight dresses, looking like I was sixteen, and drinking like I was twenty-one, with drinks purchased by men much older than that.

I paid for the meals, drinks, and parties of everyone around me so they'd be my friends. I searched for self-love and acceptance in every one of the worst possible ways. I dated the most beautiful and popular boys. When I wasn't with them, I would cheat on them with other, often older men. It was like I was starved for affection, no matter how I got it. I was in constant pursuit of feeling valuable, beautiful, and loved.

It was a dream life to anyone looking from the outside in. But inside, I was screaming for someone to shake me and tell me I was worthy of love. I wanted them to show me love, prove to me they cared about me and how I felt in a way that I could believe it, trust it ...

As it often does, the harmful fairytale lifestyle came to an end. The next ten years or so were filled with the breakdown of my family, years of feeling abandoned, a litany of addiction and total self-destruction, and eventually, being told I had "terminal" cervical cancer just one and a half years after beginning to build a real family of my own.

All I had ever wanted was a real family and a real home. I wanted somewhere I could come back to at the end of the day and feel at home. It's something I'd never had before but had seen in movies and when I would visit my friends' houses. A real home meant safety, peace, acceptance, and love.

By the time I had my beautiful daughter, Ellie, I was twenty-five and had reinvented myself more times than I could count. I had filled my body with as many poisons as I could to escape the pain, and I had been on suicide watch more than once.

To this day, I wonder if all of that contributed to me ultimately having cancer in the area where all my trauma began. But I guess I'll never have a definitive answer to that question.

The Diagnosis

Ellie was a year and a half old when I was diagnosed with cervical cancer. I was married to her father, Jerrod, but we had *just* decided to split up. We had a whirlwind romance, quickly got pregnant, and, as a result, were married before either of us knew each other. We argued constantly about life, infidelity, and our future. After a lot of brutal fights, rejections, betrayals, and marriage counseling sessions, we were both done. We knew we couldn't keep doing what *this* was for much longer. Our hearts weren't in it anymore.

By the time I found out, it was already advanced. I was twenty-five.

"You have a very aggressive and rare type of cancer," my doctor told me.

I wasn't scared at first. Despite a traumatic life, I still felt young and strong.

"You *are* young," my doctor agreed. "We have some excellent protocols and options. And if you are going to beat this, I recommend giving it everything we've got."

The doctor was referring to giving me the harshest but most powerful treatment in hopes of curing me. Older or less healthy people likely would have had a difficult time enduring the type of treatment they had in store for me.

I quickly agreed. The cancer diagnosis didn't feel real to me. It didn't occur to me that I wouldn't survive or that I couldn't handle treatments. "Do whatever you have to do to cure it," I agreed quickly.

Despite the endless conflict, the news of my cancer changed something in Jerrod. Instead of moving forward with a separation, he stayed. He promised he would never leave me for as long as I had cancer. I was both shocked and grateful to Jerrod for that. It meant that Ellie would be taken care of when I couldn't and that I didn't need to worry about finding somewhere else to live while going through treatment. It was one less thing to worry about. I wondered if this meant he was going to be there just for Ellie or if this was a real turning point, and he would be there as the husband I had always hoped for.

The doctors set up an aggressive schedule and I got started right away.

I received the most radiation I could handle and the strongest chemotherapy they could offer. That meant three different types of chemo at the same time—carboplatin, carbotaxol, and fluorouracil (or 5FU for short). Some say it's FU because of what you'd like to say to it and how much it kicks your ass (and the cancer's ass, which is a good thing).

I had twenty-eight days of radiation plus the 5FU every third week. I remember being the first to arrive at the cancer center in the morning, and the last to leave. I would watch others come and go as I surrendered to the medication and care of my doctors. We only stopped when tests showed that my levels were too low to continue and I needed a break. Even then, there were times when my doctor would beg me to put my treatment on pause to give myself some rest, but I would refuse. I felt awful, but I wanted to be cured.

My entire life, I could look at just about any problem and figure it out. My bosses at my jobs where I built their brands and their sales would say, "If there's a problem that can't be solved, give it to CoCo. She will figure it out." And I was proud of that. My entire family was entrepreneurial and the apple didn't fall far from the tree.

But this was the biggest problem I had ever faced. I accepted help. I needed it. My sister came to my side to support me and help with Ellie. She put her life on hold for a moment to take over mine. I will never be able to fully express how grateful to her I am. My mother-in-law spent more and more time with my daughter. We talked several times about how important she would be to Ellie if I were to pass away. My mother came to bolster my resolve when the effects of treatment were really bad. She was a tough woman and she tried to lend her strength to me, despite a decade of mother-daughter arguments and pain.

Until cancer, I wasn't used to accepting help of any kind, especially not from my mother. But if you're reading this, you probably already know that cancer changes everything.

I was set on being cured no matter what. I learned to advocate for myself within the medical system and with insurance companies.

Let me just say right now that I have wonderful doctors. There were times when they were right to tell me to put things on pause. But I just wanted it to be over and to be cured. I was having some awful side effects of radiation, but when I asked my radiation oncologist about it, he looked at me—I came in wearing make-up, a cute outfit, accessories—and he assumed I was exaggerating.

"If you were sick, you wouldn't look like you do right now," he said, doubtfully. I don't remember if he even did any scans. He simply disregarded my symptoms and judged me based on the fact that I hid my pain well instead of what I was telling him.

Unbeknownst to me, I was being severely burned on the inside by his negligence. The rest of my cancer care team was unaware that anything was wrong with my radiation treatment.

A couple of days later, I was at home, feeling sicker than I had ever felt before, and I was hit with a huge wave of dread and pain. I *knew* something was very wrong, but I didn't know what.

Pathetic

I woke up feeling nauseated. I was in my bedroom at the time; Jerrod and I slept in separate bedrooms by then but had agreed to live apart, yet together. I hated it but I knew it was best for Ellie. I was on heavy medications and it was a constant battle to simply stay awake.

I tried to keep from vomiting until I made it to the bathroom but my legs didn't seem to work anymore. I slid off the bed and crawled to the waste paper basket where I threw up, mostly in the basket but partially on myself.

I felt *so* sick.

Even though I was light-headed, I felt compelled to go to the kitchen for a replacement garbage bag and clean myself up. Somehow I got my legs to carry me at least to the kitchen before I ended up getting dizzy and crashing to the floor. I can still remember how much it hurt my knees, which were so bony then, to be on the hardwood floor.

I knew Jerrod hated it when my illness or existence woke him up, but I didn't have a phone and I needed an ambulance. I had no choice but to call for him.

Most days I felt as if Jerrod despised me. That night, he was determined to prove me right.

When Jerrod appeared in the kitchen doorway, I said, "Call 9-1-1. Something's wrong."

"You woke me up," he growled, looking at me on the floor.

I could feel every vibrating nerve in my body telling me I was in serious trouble.

Jerrod either didn't believe me or, much like my radiation oncologist, he didn't care.

"Oh my god, Jay, who cares about your sleep? Just please call an ambulance! Call NOW!" Did he think I was making it all up? Being dramatic? I often wonder to this day if I was so delirious with pain that I was only screaming for help in my head, and not out loud at all?! That would explain *a lot*.

Whether it was in my mind or reality, I could've sworn I heard him say, "You're *pathetic*."

I must have looked crazy, crawling around on the floor and moaning and crying with pain.

"Some of us have to sleep and go to work in the morning," he said. And with that, he turned off the kitchen lights and went back to bed.

Whether anyone believed me or not, I knew then that if I couldn't make it to my phone and call 9-1-1, I would die. I managed to crawl back far enough to get my phone.

I barely even remember doing it, but I managed to call the ambulance. Once the EMTs arrived, they began trying to find a pulse. My blood pressure was so low that they were having a hard time stabilizing me enough to make the trip to the hospital. Once they got levels to a point where they thought I might survive the five-mile ride, I was placed on a gurney.

Just that movement had me scream out in pain.

I couldn't say or do much but I remember grabbing Jerrod's hand in panic and begging him to come to the hospital with me: "Please come, Jerrod. I don't want to die alone," I whispered.

Jerrod promised he would. He told me, "I'm just going to get dressed and I'll be right behind you."

As the EMTs loaded me into the ambulance, I passed out.

Thank God for Big Miracles

I woke up in the ER with a flurry of concerned doctors and nurses rushing around me. They didn't know what was wrong. I just lay there as they ran tests and called doctors from various specialties to look at me.

After about four hours in the ER, Jerrod came in, freshly bathed, dressed, and holding a coffee he had picked up from somewhere along the way to the hospital.

I eventually was admitted to the ICU. I was vomiting uncontrollably and had constant diarrhea. What's worse, everything coming out of me was pure black. Once the doctors realized what was happening, they told me that what was coming out of me was, in fact, the burnt, radiated—essentially cremated—remains of my organs.

I was dying. That's what they said. The doctors were horrified at the extent of my radiation damage. They estimated that I had no more than six or so hours to live.

It was COVID-19 times so patients weren't allowed to have guests. But I was about to die, and I begged them to let me see my daughter. They made an exception by allowing me to see Ellie for fifteen minutes so that I could say goodbye.

How do you wrap up a lifetime's worth of love, memories, and advice for the future in fifteen minutes?

This was the first time I prayed. Truly prayed. For many reasons before this, I was not religious. My sister, who was always praying for me and leaving prayer messages around my house for healing and strength was the religious one in the family. But I always just rolled my eyes at the messages. I loved her for them, but I didn't give them a second thought otherwise. After all, what kind of God lets his children be raped at age five?

I didn't give prayers a second thought, that is, until now. At this moment, I turned to God.

Please let me stay alive until Ellie gets here. Give me more time to say all the things she needs to hear. Give me more time to live. Let me make up for my mistakes. I promise I will if you give me this.

And I *did* survive until Ellie came. I took her into my arms as best as I could and told her I'd always be in her heart and that she should always speak up for herself. I told her a lot of the things I wish someone had told me at that age. Once she left, I continued to pray. Six hours later, the beeps on the monitor evened out, my blood pressure came up, and I stabilized enough to have emergency surgery. I had been given the chance to live that I was desperate for.

I had asked—no, begged—for a miracle. And I was given one. It was an opportunity I had never imagined could truly be possible. And I have prayed every day since.

New Normal

I grew up in an environment where beauty was *everything*. Without beauty, I was worthless. And for most of my life, I agreed with that. My body had brought me nothing but pain and trauma. It had been used and treated like garbage. It had been dressed beautifully but was rotten beneath.

I woke up from an eight-hour life-saving surgery and realized *I was alive!* It seemed impossible. Less than one day earlier, I was saying my final goodbye to my beautiful little girl. And now I was here: awake, alive, and breathing.

I immediately thanked God for listening to my prayers. I am sure I said hundreds of prayers of thanks and gratefulness in mere seconds.

As the shock wore off, my surroundings came into view, and the surgery pain started to settle in. I realized my life had changed.

I looked down from my elevated hospital bed to see this thing attached to me. I soon learned that it was my ostomy bag. I could feel the ache of a huge incision and the gauze that covered it. I felt the pull and pain of multiple objects pulling on my back. These would end up being my nephrostomy tubes.

I had a port coming out of my chest and monitors all around me. One of the doctors explained that due to damage or disease of my intestines, kidneys, and other organs, they had to give me a loop ileostomy and replace my damaged ureters with tubes leading to bags. My surgeon, Dr. Paul Gray, and his team told me they'd never seen radiation damage as bad as they saw when they operated on me. My organs, intestines, all of it, were burned inside and out.

This was my new normal.

At first, I didn't have the freedom to worry about what I looked like. My body had been the source of my pain my whole life. This was just a different kind of pain. My appearance wasn't on my radar.

My care team kept me focused on learning how to function. This included learning how to eat, sleep, and even walk. And it included how to handle my new mobility aids—which is exactly what ostomy and nephrostomy bags are. They're no different than needing a wheelchair to move or an oxygen tank to breathe.

I could see myself in the way that Jerrod looked at me the first time he walked into my hospital room. His eyes went directly to my bags and then darted away. His face filled with sadness and disgust (or was it fear?). He was the person who was supposed to love me in sickness and in health, and he couldn't even look at me. Bags, tubes, and all.

Despite our constant fighting and near-divorce, I did and still do have an idea of how scary it all must have looked. I was terrified too. Jerrod admitted he would rather die than go through a cancer battle like the one I was going through. It was an awful thing to say, but if someone had told me a couple of years beforehand that this would be my journey, there's no way I could've imagined getting through it.

When I talked to my mom about how Jerrod's face had made me sad and angry, rejected again, she gently suggested that I just stay with him. In her mind, she couldn't see a way for me to be with anyone else now that I had bags and cancer and all the rest of it. I guess now, I didn't just come with baggage—I came with actual bags. After all, my mother, like my sister and I, had been judged based on her appearance for most of her life. She wasn't trying to be hurtful. But her words made me hate myself just a little bit more nonetheless.

Here's the thing … You have no idea what you're capable of doing until you're forced to do it. At first, I couldn't look in the mirror. I had to fight not to be horrified by the look of my bags.

But then, I started thanking God for them. They saved my life. I made it my mission to make sure everyone close to me knew that too.

I have always turned to makeup and fashion to make me feel better. But after the surgery, beauty wasn't on my radar. At one point, I even donated all of my pre-cancer clothing, thinking I would never be able to wear something that looked good again.

For the first time in my life, I didn't do my makeup or hair. I just focused on recovering. I pretty much lived in Jerrod's XXL clothes.

I spent months in a hospital bed, connected to IVs and monitors, tubes, and bags. I was alone most of the time. Jerrod tried to visit as much as he could, but they were often awkward, sometimes angry, visits. I could see that the longer my cancer journey was drawn out, the more resentment was building within Jerrod. On the other hand, he brought bring Ellie to see me. Her visits were my everything. I used her visits as fuel for motivation to keep going and to fight. She was my inspiration for not giving up. She was my reason for focusing on staying alive.

On good days, we would walk through the hospital and go to the vending machine. On other days, she would curl up on me and cuddle. We would watch movies on her iPad, talk, and giggle together.

As I spent more and more time in the hospital, I began sharing more and more of my story on Instagram and watched as people everywhere started following along. I aimed for complete transparency. I would go live from the hospital at all hours of the day and night. I was essentially trapped in my bed and had to learn how to walk, empty my bags, and function as a human being all over again. So between visits from my sister and Ellie, it was my online community of CoCo Strong followers that kept me going.

I had been brought up to hide anything that wasn't perfect and beautiful about me. But there were over 100,000 people who strangely loved me despite the bags and the lack of makeup. Even better, they loved me for the fact that I was being real. This was the first time I realized just how many others are just as broken as I was. The community filled up with people who were also going through cancer or who had just gone through it, with people who were dealing with ostomies, tubes, or drains, and with those who were just looking to feel like they weren't alone in this world, no matter what their journey looked like.

For the first time, I realized what my purpose was. I started to see myself differently. I realized that everything I had been through, all of the traumatic events of my childhood and afterward, had led to this moment. They had made me strong enough to endure my treatments while helping others.

Having a true purpose saved me. Learning that I was worthy of love saved me. Having the chance to spend more time with Ellie saved me.

I found that things got much better once I could take care of myself. I can clean and empty my ostomy bag in seconds. I have found the perfect stretchy shorts to wear over and tuck up into my nephrostomy bags so that they're not hanging out below my shorts. Oh. And I can wear shorts again! And tank tops, believe it or not. Nothing shows when I do except for maybe the top oval part of the seal of my ostomy. Or the bandage over the top of it and my incision.

I'm not going to lie. I have had several horrible spills since getting my bags, especially in the beginning. And don't get me started on splashback when trying to empty a bag in a public toilet! But no matter what, I simply tell whoever I'm with that I've gotta go. I head back home, clean myself up, and start over. I have become good at this. And I'm good at preventing it from happening in the first place. I know what to eat and what not to because certain foods go through my intestines faster than others.

Knowing all of this helps me stay out longer without having any ostomy explosions or leaks. With more time and more predictability, I am more confident when I'm out of the house. I can take Ellie and my dog Bruno to the Starbucks drive-through for pup cups and cake pops without unwanted surprises.

I'll admit that I've had some near-death emergencies since my six-hours-to-live event. But I'm still here. I spend roughly thirty percent of my life in the hospital due to infections, tube changes, and other procedures. I have a palliative care team I love. I have a doctor who I can text when I feel an infection coming on so that we don't waste time waiting before we jump on it. I know now that time matters. Everything matters. Any delays in care or listening to my body's cues that something is wrong cost me my health and the time I have to spend with the people I love.

I know everything there is to know about my medications and care needs. I don't waste time trying to explain my entire case to ER doctors. I just point them to my file or have my palliative care doctor call them. I advocate for myself when I need to. I am a favorite patient to most of the nurses on the floor they usually set me up in. My cancer care team and I talk real talk. We celebrate when we can and we cry together when we have to. I order pizza for everyone on the floor on busy nights to pick up everyone's spirits, and I do as much of this as I can in between viral video posts and live events with those who have come to rely on me for inspiration and advice.

I can look in the mirror now. I do my makeup regularly. I get my nails done. I do all the things I need to to feel beautiful.

I have learned how to live with *and love* my bags. They are tiny miracles attached to my body. I now know how to dress in clothes that make me feel cute. And if living this way means that I occasionally have to empty my ostomy bag into a ditch on the side of the road in an emergency, so be it. It's worth it.

I cherish each moment that I'm not in hospital, but I also cherish the ones when I am. Because I'm alive. And I have a purpose that matters.

Self-Love at Last

I have suffered more trauma than anyone should ever have to. I know that. I know it broke me from a very young age. I know I've made massive mistakes and hurt the people I love. But I also know that all of that—all of the pain and heartache—*that* is what made me strong enough to persevere through my cancer journey.

I look at everything differently now. I look at *me* differently now.

I love my mistakes and the difficult ways in which I've had to learn them. They have made me humble, grateful, and wise.

I love my bags. They keep my feet on this earth to dance with my daughter, pray with my sister, and slowly begin to heal my relationship with my mom. My bags make it so that I can travel to Miami to spend time with my core family. They have allowed me to host in-person events where I share my full story with people who love me and, in those moments and spaces, feel so completely accepted and loved that it's hard to find the right words to describe it.

They give me the ability to focus my energy on fulfilling my purpose by sharing more and more of my story with the people who find healing and support from it.

(And yes, Jerrod and I are still together; even though our marriage is more broken now than ever. I'm not sure what the future holds for us, but I'm not going to use what time I have left on this earth being angry or hurt by the man who completely disregards the strength it has taken and the challenges I've endured just to be here.)

Most of all, I love *myself*, for the first time in my life. I embrace the quiet, I see the beauty of life's details, and I'm proud to be an example of resilience to so many.

It's cancer that has led me to this point. Without it, I don't think I'd be here to tell my story today.

And that's why I'll always say, cancer has saved my life.

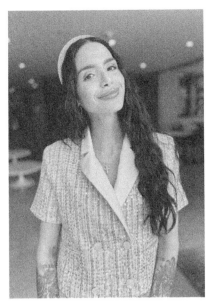

NICOLE "COCO" ROPER

Nicole "CoCo" Roper is a motivational speaker, life coach, cancer hero, and disability advocate. By being painfully transparent about her journey with cancer, CoCo draws people into her world, online and in person.

She shares everything, good or bad, with a community of over 100,000 followers on Instagram and TikTok. CoCo also speaks at sold-out events such as 'Coffee with CoCo' and motivational workshops designed to inspire people to happiness.

CoCo built six and seven-figure fashion brands before her cancer diagnosis. Despite a traumatic personal life, CoCo has proven to be a brilliant entrepreneur whose CoCoStrong brand stands for resilience against all odds, both in the USA and Costa Rica.

CoCo inspires others to love themselves and embrace their difficult journeys. Her book, *Look at Me*, which details her life of trauma, resiliency, love, loss, and profound purpose, is scheduled to hit shelves in February 2024. To be notified when it is published, visit her on Instagram.

Follow her on social media for more of CoCo's story.

Instagram & TikTok: @IAMCOCOSTRONG

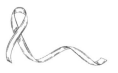

CHAPTER FOUR

MÍRAME

por CoCo Roper

Puede que solo tenga veintinueve años, pero ya he vivido muchas vidas diferentes. Sorprendentemente, es *esta* vida, la infiltrada por el cáncer, las cirugías, las bolsas de discapacidad y la lucha por mi vida, la que me salvó.

Vengo de una familia que siempre ha estado en el punto de mira. Para las personas, éramos como la versión costarricense de las Kardashian. Mi madre siempre estuvo en el punto de mira. Era puertorriqueña, guapísima y de la alta sociedad. En los años 90, incluso fue coronada Miss Puerto Rico. Sus esposos y toda nuestra familia han aparecido en innumerables revistas de noticias y entretenimiento puertorriqueñas y costarricenses a lo largo de nuestras vidas. Esto se debe a que la gente estaba deslumbrada por el glamour, la moda, la fama y el dinero que nos rodeaba, y el drama, por supuesto.

A pesar de tener fanáticos que seguían cada uno de nuestros movimientos como familia, los extraños solo veían alrededor del 10 por ciento de la realidad de nuestras vidas fracturadas.

Cuando tenía cuatro años y medio, mi madre se divorció de mi padre biológico. Su matrimonio había sido inestable en el mejor de los casos. Mi padre le había exigido a mi madre que renunciara a mucho de lo que amaba, como modelar, trabajar en televisión y construir su marca, para ser una madre que se quedara en casa y una esposa ideal para él. Su matrimonio estaba destinado al fracaso. Y cuando sucedió, comenzó mi pesadilla.

Veía a mi padre biológico durante dos días cada dos semanas después de que se separaran. En estas visitas, seríamos una verdadera familia durante el día. Mi hermana, mi medio hermano, mi papá y yo nos perseguíamos por la amplia propiedad en cuadraciclos, hacíamos parrilladas y nadábamos en la piscina, e incluso bebíamos alcohol, esto siendo aún menores de edad. Sobre todo, pasábamos tiempo juntos como una familia, que es todo lo que cualquier niño quisiera.

Pero por la noche, las cosas cambiaban, para mí y mi hermana (aunque no lo sabía en ese momento). Desde los cinco años, mi padre biológico abusó sexualmente de mí. Y eso me quebró de una manera que jamás pude imaginar posible. Nunca me tocó mientras estaba con mi mamá. Pero una vez que se divorciaron, fue una tortura. Esto continuó hasta que cumplí nueve años y tuve mi menstruación, gracias a Dios que la tuve antes que la mayoría de las otras niñas.

Converso mucho más de ello en mi libro "Mírame", pero por ahora, trata de entender que mi abuso marcó el comienzo, de una incapacidad permanente para amarme a mí misma o a mi cuerpo de una manera saludable. Esto condujo a una vida de autodestrucción, dolor, adicción y reinvención. Incluso, de alguna manera, puede haberme llevado a mi cáncer.

Increíblemente, cuando no estaba en la casa de mi padre, vivía una vida de cuento de hadas. Dejaba de lado todo lo que sucedía en el fin de semana y vivía una vida llena de magia. A mis 6 años mi mamá se casó con Gary, quien se convirtió en mi padrastro. Y yo lo adoraba, era un papa increíble. Tenía más dinero del que mi madre, mi hermana o yo habíamos visto en la vida real. Estaba en todas partes. Pero yo lo amaba por lo especial que era con nosotros. El amor que nos daba que en realidad nunca había recibido de una figura paterna. Teníamos sirvientas, guardaespaldas, ventanas enrejadas (para nuestra protección) y vehículos blindados. Nos vigilaban dondequiera que íbamos. No había privacidad. Cada movimiento, evento o error que cometíamos corría el riesgo de ser exagerado y vinculado con nuestra madre. Eso significaba que nuestras vidas exigían belleza, perfección y vestimenta de clase alta. A los diez años, llevaba tacones de Burberry y bolsos Louis Vuitton. Cuando tenía once o doce años, estaba en bares, con vestidos ajustados, como si tuviera dieciséis, bebiendo como si tuviera veintiuno, con bebidas compradas por hombres mucho mayores que yo.

Pagué las comidas, las bebidas y las fiestas de todos los que me rodeaban para que fueran mis amigos. Busqué el amor propio y la aceptación de la peor manera posible. Salí con los chicos más guapos y populares. Cuando no estaba con ellos, les era infiel con otros hombres, a menudo mayores. Era como si estuviera hambrienta por cariño, sin importar cómo lo obtuviera.

Estaba en búsqueda constantemente de sentirme valiosa, hermosa y amada.

Era una vida de ensueño para cualquiera que mirara desde afuera hacia adentro. Pero por dentro, gritaba para que alguien me sacudiera y me dijera que era digna de amor. Quería que me mostraran amor, que me demostraran que se preocupaban por mí y por cómo me sentía de una manera que pudiera creerlo, confiar que así era ...

Como suele suceder, el dañino estilo de vida de cuento de hadas llegó a su fin. Los siguientes diez años más o menos estuvieron llenos de la desintegración de mi familia, años de sentirme abandonada, una cadena de adicción y autodestrucción total, y finalmente, me dijeron que tenía cáncer cervical "terminal" solo un año y medio después de comenzar a construir mi propia verdadera familia.

Todo lo que siempre había querido era una familia y un hogar real. Quería un lugar al que pudiera volver al final del día y sentirme en casa. Es algo que nunca había tenido antes, pero que había visto en películas y cuando visitaba las casas de mis amigos. Un verdadero hogar significaba seguridad, paz, aceptación y amor.

Cuando tuve a mi hermosa hija, Ellie, tenía veinticinco años y ya me había reinventado más veces de las que podía contar. Había llenado mi cuerpo con tantos venenos como pude para escapar del dolor, y había estado bajo vigilancia de suicidio más de una vez.

Hasta el día de hoy, me pregunto si todo eso contribuyó a que finalmente tuviera cáncer en el área donde comenzó todo mi trauma. Pero supongo que nunca tendré una respuesta definitiva a esa pregunta.

El Diagnóstico

Mi hija, Ellie, tenía un año y medio cuando me diagnosticaron cáncer de cuello uterino. Yo estaba casada con su padre, Jerrod, pero acabábamos de decidir separarnos. Tuvimos un romance relámpago, rápidamente quedé embarazada y, como resultado, nos casamos antes de que ninguno de los dos nos conociéramos completamente. Discutíamos constantemente; sobre la vida, la infidelidad y nuestro futuro. Después de muchas peleas brutales, rechazos, traiciones y sesiones de consejería matrimonial, ambos nos habíamos rendido. Sabíamos que no podíamos seguir haciendo lo que era *esto* por mucho más tiempo. Nuestros corazones ya no estaban dedicados a el matrimonio.

Cuando me enteré que tenia cáncer, ya estaba avanzado. Tenía veinticinco años.

"Tienes un tipo de cáncer muy agresivo y raro", me dijo mi médico.

Al principio no tenía miedo. A pesar de una vida traumática, todavía me sentía joven y fuerte. Ya había superado tanto en mi vida que cáncer no era algo que me causaba terror. Así de intocable me sentía.

"*Eres* joven", coincidió mi médico. "Tenemos algunos protocolos y opciones realmente buenos. Y si vas a superar esto, te recomiendo que lo tratemos todo".

El médico se refería a darme el tratamiento más fuerte pero más poderoso, con la esperanza de curarme. Las personas mayores o menos sanas probablemente habrían tenido dificultades para soportar el tipo de tratamiento que tenían reservado para mí.

Acepté rápidamente. El diagnóstico de cáncer no me pareció real. No se me ocurrió que no sobreviviría o que no podría soportar los tratamientos. "Haz lo que tengas que hacer para curarlo", acepté rápidamente.

A pesar del interminable conflicto, la noticia de mi cáncer cambió algo en Jerrod. En lugar de seguir adelante con una separación, decidimos quedarnos juntos. Me prometió que nunca me dejaría mientras tuviera cáncer. Estaba sorprendida y agradecida con Jerrod por eso. Esto significaba que Ellie sería atendida y amada cuando yo no pudiera y que no tenía que preocuparme por encontrar otro lugar para vivir mientras pasaba por el tratamiento. Era una cosa menos de la que tenia preocuparse y me daba lo oportunidad de enfocarme 100% en combatir el cáncer. Me pregunté a mi misma si esto significaba que iba a estar allí solo para Ellie o si este era un verdadero punto de inflexión, y él estaría allí como el esposo que siempre había esperado.

Los médicos establecieron un horario agresivo de tratamiento y comencé de inmediato.En una semana y media mi vida había cambiado drásticamente.

Recibí la mayor cantidad de radiación que pude soportar y la quimioterapia más fuerte que pudieron ofrecerme. Eso significaba tres tipos diferentes de quimioterapia al mismo tiempo; carboplatino, carbotaxol y fluorouracilo (o 5FU para abreviar). Algunos le dicen FU por lo que te gustaría decirle y lo mucho que te patea el trasero (y el trasero del cáncer, lo cual es algo bueno).

Recibí veintiocho sesiones de radiación más la quimioterapia cada tres semanas. Recuerdo ser la primera en llegar al centro oncológico por la mañana y la última en irme. Veía a otros ir y venir mientras yo me rendía a la medicación y al cuidado de mis médicos. Solo nos detuviamos cuando las pruebas mostraron que mis niveles eran demasiado bajos para continuar y necesitaba un descanso. Incluso, hubieron momentos en los que mi médico me rogaba que pusiera mi tratamiento en pausa para descansar un poco, pero me negaba. Me sentía fatal, pero quería curarme. Ya quería terminar y seguir con mi vida.

Toda mi vida, pude ver casi cualquier problema y "resolverlo". Mis jefes en mis trabajos, donde construí sus marcas y sus ventas, decían: "Si hay un problema que no se puede resolver, dáselo a CoCo. Ella lo resolverá". Y estaba orgullosa de eso. Toda mi familia era emprendedora y la manzana no caía lejos del árbol.

Pero este era el mayor problema al que me había enfrentado. Tuve que aceptar ayuda. La necesitaba mas que nunca. Mi hermana vino a mi lado para apoyarme y ayudar con Ellie. Puso su vida en pausa por un largo tiempo para encargarse de la mía. Nunca podré expresar completamente lo agradecida que estoy con ella. Mi suegra pasaba cada vez más tiempo con mi hija. Hablamos varias veces sobre lo importante que sería para mi que ella estuviera apoyando a Ellie de la mejor manera, si yo falleciera.

Mi mama vino a reforzar mi determinación cuando los efectos del tratamiento eran realmente malos. Era una mujer fuerte y trató de prestarme su resiliencia, a pesar de una década de discusiones y dolor entre madre e hija.

Hasta el cáncer, no estaba acostumbrada a aceptar ayuda de ningún tipo, especialmente de mi madre. Pero si estás leyendo esto, probablemente ya sepas que el cáncer lo cambia todo.

Estaba decidida a curarme pasara lo que pasara. Aprendí a abogar por mí misma dentro del sistema médico y con las compañías de seguros.

Permítanme decir ahora mismo que tengo médicos maravillosos. Hubo momentos en los que tenían razón al decirme que pusiera las cosas en pausa. Pero yo solo quería terminar y curarme. Estaba teniendo algunos efectos secundarios terribles de la radiación, pero cuando le pregunté a mi oncólogo radioterapeuta al respecto, me miró a través de una llamada virtual, llegué con maquillaje, un atuendo lindo, accesorios, y asumió que estaba exagerando.

"Si estuvieras enferma, no te verías como te ves ahora", dijo, dubitativo. Simplemente ignoró mis síntomas, juzgándome por el hecho de que ocultaba bien mi dolor, en lugar de lo que le estaba diciendo.

Sin que yo lo supiera, estaba sufriendo graves quemaduras en el interior por su negligencia. Y el resto de mi equipo de atención médica contra el cáncer no sabía que algo andaba mal con mi tratamiento de radiación.

Un par de días después estaba en casa, sintiéndome más enferma que nunca, y fui golpeada por una gran ola de temor y dolor. *Sabía* que algo andaba muy mal, pero no sabía qué.

Patético

Me desperté sintiendo náuseas. Yo estaba en mi habitación en ese momento; Para entonces, Jerrod y yo dormíamos en habitaciones separadas, habíamos acordado vivir juntos, pero separados. Detestaba vivir asi, pero sabía que era lo mejor para Ellie. Tomaba medicamentos sumamente fuertes y era una batalla constante simplemente mantenerme despierta. Traté de no vomitar hasta que llegué al baño, pero mis piernas ya no parecían funcionar. Me deslicé de la cama y me arrastré hasta el basurero donde vomité, sobre todo en el basurero y parcialmente sobre mí misma. Me sentí *muy* mal. Peor de lo que jamás había pensado posible. Debil, mareada, adolorida, con vomito en mis pantalones y frio en mi cabeza ya que había perdido todo mi pelo de la quimioterapia.

A pesar de que estaba mareada, me sentí obligada a ir a la cocina por una bolsa de basura de reemplazo y limpiarme. De alguna manera conseguí que mis piernas me llevaran al menos a la cocina antes de que terminara mareándome y estrellándome contra el suelo en las escaleras y termine en el piso de mi cuarto golpeándome la cadera de mi cuerpo tan frágil.

Sabía que Jerrod odiaba cuando mi enfermedad o mi existencia lo despertaban, pero yo no tenía teléfono y necesitaba una ambulancia. No tuve más remedio que llamarlo.

La mayoría de los días sentía como si Jerrod me despreciara. Esa noche, estaba decidido a darme la razón.

Cuando Jerrod apareció en la puerta de la cocina, le dije: "Llama al 9-1-1. Algo anda mal".

—Me has despertado —gruñó, mirándome en el suelo—.

Podía sentir cada nervio vibrante de mi cuerpo diciéndome que estaba en serios problemas. Jerrod no me creyó o, al igual que mi oncólogo radioterapeuta, no le importó.

"Oh, Dios mío, Jay, ¿a quién le importa tu sueño? ¡Por favor, llama a una ambulancia! ¡Llama AHORA!" ¿Pensó que me lo estaba inventando todo? ¿Era un drama? A menudo me pregunto hasta el día de hoy si yo estaba delirando de tanto dolor que solo gritaba pidiendo ayuda en mi cabeza, y no en voz alta. Eso explicaría *muchas cosas.*

Ya sea en mi mente o en la realidad, podría haber jurado que lo escuché decir: "Eres *patética.*"

Debo haber parecido loca, arrastrándome por el suelo y gimiendo y llorando de dolor. Todavía recuerdo lo mucho que me dolían las rodillas (que en ese entonces eran tan huesudas) de la perdida de peso tan drástica que había tenido por el tratamiento.

"Algunos de nosotros tenemos que dormir e ir a trabajar por la mañana", dijo. Y con eso, apagó las luces de la cocina y volvió a la cama.

Ya sea que alguien me creyera o no, *supe* entonces que si no podía llegar a mi teléfono y llamar al 9-1-1, moriría. Me las arreglé para arrastrarme lo suficiente como para coger mi teléfono.

Apenas recuerdo haberlo hecho, pero logré llamar a la ambulancia.

Una vez que llegaron los paramédicos, comenzaron a tratar de encontrarme el pulso. Mi presión arterial era tan baja que estaban teniendo dificultades para estabilizarme lo suficiente como para hacer el viaje al hospital. Una vez que llegaron a un punto en el que pensaron que podría sobrevivir al viaje de cinco millas, me colocaron en una camilla.

No podía decir ni hacer mucho, pero recuerdo que agarré la mano de Jerrod con pánico y le supliqué que viniera conmigo al hospital. —Por favor, ven, Jerrod. No quiero morir sola, tengo miedo —susurré—.

Jerrod prometió que lo haría. Me dijo: "Me voy a vestir y estaré justo detrás de ti y la ambulancia".

Cuando los paramédicos me subieron a la ambulancia, me desmayé.

Gracias a Dios por los Grandes Milagros

Me desperté en la sala de emergencias con una ráfaga de médicos y enfermeras preocupados corriendo a mi alrededor. No sabían qué pasaba. Me quedé allí acostada llena de pánico sin tener la menor idea de que estaba pasando, mientras me hacían pruebas y llamaban a médicos de varias especialidades para que me vieran.

Después de unas cuatro horas en la sala de emergencias, Jerrod entró, recién bañado, vestido y sosteniendo un café que había recogido en algún lugar de camino al hospital.

Finalmente me ingresaron en la UCI. Vomitaba incontrolablemente y tenía diarrea constante. Lo que es peor, todo lo que salía de mí era negro puro.

Una vez que los médicos se dieron cuenta de lo que estaba pasando, me dijeron que lo que salía de mí eran en realidad los restos quemados, irradiados, básicamente incinerados, de mis órganos y tejido.

Me estaba muriendo. Eso es lo que dijeron. Los médicos estaban horrorizados por la magnitud de mi daño por radiación. Calcularon que no me quedaban más de seis horas de vida.

Eran tiempos de COVID-19, por lo que a los pacientes no se les permitía tener visitas. Pero estaba a punto de morir y les rogué que me dejaran ver a mi hija. Hicieron una excepción al permitirme ver a Ellie durante quince minutos para que pudiera despedirme.

¿Cómo se resume toda una vida de amor, recuerdos y consejos para el futuro en quince minutos?

Esta fue la primera vez que oré. Verdaderamente orar. Por muchas razones antes de esto, yo no era religiosa ni creía en el poder de Dios. Mi hermana, que siempre estaba orando por mí y dejando mensajes de oración en mi casa para sanar y fortalecerme, era la religiosa de la familia. Pero yo, siempre ponía los ojos en blanco ante los mensajes. La amaba por ellos, pero ni los pensé dos veces,. Después de todo, ¿qué clase de Dios permite que sus hijos sean violados a los cinco años?

No pensé dos veces en las oraciones, al menos hasta ahora. En ese momento recurrí a Dios. *Por favor, déjame seguir con vida hasta que Ellie llegue. Dame más tiempo para decirle todas las cosas que necesita escuchar. Dame más tiempo de vida. Permíteme enmendar mis errores. Te prometo que lo haré si me das este priviliegio.*

Y sobreviví hasta que *llegó* Ellie. La tomé en mis brazos lo mejor que pude y le dije que siempre estaría en su corazón y que siempre debería hablar por sí misma. Le conté muchas de las cosas que me hubiera gustado que alguien me hubiera dicho a esa edad. Una vez que se fue, seguí orando. No paraba de llorar de la tristeza de que jamás volvería a ver a mi hija. El dolor emocional era mas fuerte que el dolor físico. Seis horas más tarde, los pitidos en el monitor se nivelaron, mi presión arterial subió y me estabilicé lo suficiente como para soportar una cirugía de emergencia. Dios me había dado la oportunidad de vivir por la que estaba desesperada. Había pedido, suplicado, un milagro. Y me dieron uno. Era una oportunidad que nunca había imaginado que pudiera ser realmente posible. Era un milagro que no podía ignorar. Y por primera vez vi el poder de la oración y de Dios. Y he orado todos los días desde entonces.

Nueva Normalidad

Crecí en un ambiente donde la belleza lo era *todo*. Sin belleza, no valía nada. Y durante la mayor parte de mi vida, estuve de acuerdo con eso. Mi cuerpo no me había traído nada más que dolor y trauma. Había sido usado y tratado como basura, primordialmente por mi misma.. Había sido vestido maravillosamente, pero estaba podrido por debajo.

¡Me desperté de una cirugía de ocho horas que *me salvó la vida*! Parecía imposible. Menos de un día antes, le estaba dando el último adiós a mi hermosa niña. Y ahora estaba aquí: despierta, viva, respirando.

Inmediatamente le di gracias a Dios por escuchar mis oraciones. Estoy segura de que dije cientos de oraciones de agradecimiento en cuestión de segundos.

A medida que el asombro pasaba, mi entorno quedó a la vista y el dolor de la cirugía comenzó a asentarse. Me di cuenta de que mi vida había cambiado.

Miré hacia abajo desde mi cama elevada de hospital y vi esta cosa adherida a mí. Pronto supe que era mi bolsa de ostomía. Podía sentir el dolor de una enorme incisión y la gasa que la cubría. Sentí el golpe y el dolor de múltiples objetos tirando de mi espalda.

Estos terminarían siendo mis tubos de nefrostomía.

Tenía un caterer que salía de mi pecho y monitores a mi alrededor.

Uno de los médicos me explicó que, debido a un daño o enfermedad de mis intestinos, riñones y otros órganos, tuvieron que hacerme una ileostomía y reemplazar mis uréteres dañados con tubos que conducen a bolsas. Mi cirujano, el Dr. Paul Gray, y su equipo me dijeron que nunca habían visto un daño por radiación tan grave como el que vieron cuando me operaron. Mis órganos, intestinos, todo, estaba quemado por dentro y por fuera.

Esta era mi nueva normalidad.

Al principio, no tenía la libertad de preocuparme por mi apariencia. Mi cuerpo había sido la fuente de mi dolor toda mi vida. Este era simplemente un tipo de dolor diferente. Mi apariencia no estaba en mi radar.

Mi equipo de atención me mantuvo concentrada en aprender cómo manejar mi nueva normalidad. Esto incluía aprender a comer, dormir e incluso caminar. E incluía cómo manejar mis nuevas ayudas para la movilidad, que es exactamente lo que son las bolsas de ostomía y nefrostomía. No son diferentes a necesitar una silla de ruedas para moverse o un tanque de oxígeno para respirar.

Podía verme a mí misma en la forma en que Jerrod me miró la primera vez que entró en mi habitación del hospital. Sus ojos se dirigieron directamente a mis bolsas y luego se alejaron. Su rostro estaba lleno de enojo y asco (¿o era miedo?).

Él era la persona que se suponía que debía amarme en la salud y en la enfermedad, y ni siquiera podía mirarme. Bolsas, tubos y todo. Estas bolsas y tubos eran la razón por la cual estaba viva, porque Jerrod no podía ver la belleza en eso?

A pesar de nuestras constantes peleas y casi divorcio, tenía y sigo teniendo una idea de lo aterrador que debe haber parecido todo. Yo también estaba aterrorizada. Jerrod admitió que preferiría morir antes que pasar por una batalla contra el cáncer como la que yo estaba pasando. Fue algo horrible de decir, pero si alguien me hubiera dicho un par de años antes que este sería mi viaje, no hay forma de que pudiera haber imaginado superarlo.

Cuando hablé con mi madre sobre cómo la cara de Jerrod me había puesto triste y enojada, rechazada de nuevo, ella me sugirió gentilmente que me quedara con él. En su mente, no podía ver una manera de que yo estuviera con nadie más, ahora que tenía bolsas y cáncer y todo lo demás. Supongo que ahora, no solo venia con "equipaje", pero también venia con bolsas reales. Después de todo, mi mama, al igual que mi hermana y yo, había sido juzgada por su apariencia durante la mayor parte de su vida. No estaba tratando de ser hiriente. Sin embargo, sus palabras me hicieron odiarme un poco más. Quien iba a quererme así?

Esta es la cuestión ... No tienes idea de lo que eres capaz de hacer hasta que estas obligado a hacerlo. Al principio no podía mirarme en el espejo. Tuve que luchar para no horrorizarme por el aspecto de mis bolsas.

Pero poco a poco, empecé a darle gracias a Dios por ellas. Me salvaron la vida. Me propuse asegurarme de que todas las personas cercanas a mí también lo supieran.

Siempre he recurrido al maquillaje y a la moda para sentirme mejor. Pero después de la cirugía, la belleza no estaba en mi radar. En un momento dado, incluso doné toda mi ropa pre-cáncer, pensando que nunca podría volver a usar algo que se viera bien.

Por primera vez en mi vida, no me maquillaba no me peinaba porque no tenia casi pelo. Decidí ignorar lo físico y enfocarme en la recuperación. Prácticamente vivía con la ropa XXL de Jerrod y si no estaba hospitalizada teniendo otra cirugía estaba en mi casa sola estudiando la Biblia y sanando de adentro para afuera, salir de casa no era una opción.

Pasé meses en una cama de hospital, conectada a vías intravenosas, monitores, tubos y bolsas. Si no estaba con mi hermana o mi mama, estaba sola la mayor parte del tiempo. Jerrod trató de visitar todo lo que pudo, pero a menudo eran visitas incómodas, a veces frustrantes porque solo veía el reloj para completar la hora diaria de visitar a CoCo. Pude ver que cuanto más se prolongaba mi batalla contra el cáncer, más resentimiento se acumulaba dentro de Jerrod. Por otro lado, llevaba a Ellie a verme. Sus visitas eran mi todo. Utilicé sus visitas como combustible para motivarme a seguir adelante y luchar. Ella fue, es y siempre sera mi inspiración para no rendirme. Ella fue la razón por la que me concentré en mantenerme con vida.

En los días buenos, caminábamos por el hospital e íbamos a la máquina expendedora. Otros días, se acurrucaba sobre mí y me abrazaba. Veíamos películas en su iPad, hablábamos y nos reíamos juntas.

A medida que pasaba más y más tiempo en el hospital, comencé a compartir más y más de mi historia en Instagram y vi cómo personas de todas partes empezaban a seguirme. Mi objetivo era lograr una transparencia total. Realizaba en vivos desde el hospital a todas horas del día y de la noche. Estaba prácticamente atrapada en mi cama y tuve que aprender a caminar, vaciar mis bolsas y, esencialmente, volver a funcionar como un ser humano. Entonces, entre las visitas de Ellie y mi hermana, fue mi comunidad de seguidores en línea de CoCo Strong la que me mantuvo en pie.

Me habían educado para ocultar cualquier cosa que no fuera perfecta y hermosa. Pero habían más de 100.000 personas que extrañamente me amaban a pesar de las bolsas y la falta de maquillaje. Mejor aún, me amaban por el hecho de que estaba siendo real. Esta fue la primera vez que me di cuenta de cuántos otros están tan rotos como yo. La comunidad se llenó de personas que también estaban pasando por un cáncer o que acababan de pasarlo, con personas que estaban lidiando con ostomías, tubos o drenajes, y aquellos que solo buscaban sentir que no estaban solos en este mundo, sin importar cómo fuera su viaje.

Por primera vez, me di cuenta de cuál era mi propósito. Empecé a verme de otra manera. Me di cuenta de que todo lo que había pasado, todos los eventos traumáticos de mi infancia y posteriores, me habían llevado a este momento. Me habían hecho lo suficientemente fuerte como para soportar mis tratamientos mientras ayudaba a los demás.

Tener un verdadero propósito me salvó. Aprender que yo era digna de amor me salvó. Tener la oportunidad de pasar más tiempo con Ellie me salvó.

Descubrí que las cosas mejoraron mucho una vez que pude cuidar de mí misma. Puedo limpiar y vaciar mi bolsa de ostomía en segundos. He encontrado los shorts elásticos perfectos para usar y meterlos en mis bolsas de nefrostomía para que no cuelguen debajo de mis shorts. Oh. ¡Y pude volver a usar shorts y amisetas sin mangas, lo creas o no! No se ve nada cuando lo hago, excepto tal vez la parte ovalada superior del sello de mi ostomía. O el vendaje sobre ella y mi incisión.

No voy a mentir. He tenido varios derrames horribles desde que recibí mis bolsas, especialmente al principio. ¡Y no me hagas hablar de salpicaduras al intentar vaciar una bolsa en un baño público! Pero pase lo que pase, simplemente le digo a quien sea con quien esté que tengo que irme. Regreso a casa, me limpio y empiezo de nuevo. Me he vuelto buena en esto. Y en primer lugar soy buena evitando que esto suceda. Sé qué comer y qué no porque ciertos alimentos pasan por mis intestinos más rápido que otros.

Saber todo esto me ayuda a permanecer fuera más tiempo sin tener explosiones o fugas de ostomía. Con más tiempo y más prevención, tengo más confianza cuando estoy fuera de casa. Puedo llevar a Ellie y a mi perro Bruno al autoservicio de Starbucks para comprar tazas para cachorros y cake pops sin sorpresas no deseadas.

Admito que he tenido algunas emergencias cercanas a la muerte desde mi evento de seis horas de vida. Pero sigo aquí. Paso aproximadamente el treinta por ciento de mi vida en el hospital debido a infecciones, cambios de tubos y otros procedimientos. Tengo un equipo de cuidados paliativos que me encanta. Tengo un médico al que puedo enviar mensajes de texto cuando siento que se avecina una infección para que no perdamos el tiempo esperando antes de atacarla. Ahora sé que el tiempo importa. Todo importa. Cualquier retraso en la atención o ignorar las señales de mi cuerpo de que algo anda mal me puede costar mi salud y el tiempo que tengo para pasar con las personas que amo.

Sé todo lo que hay que saber sobre mis medicamentos y necesidades de atención. No pierdo el tiempo tratando de explicar todo mi caso a los médicos de urgencias. Simplemente les señalo mi expediente o le pido a mi médico de cuidados paliativos que los llame. Me defiendo a mí misma cuando lo necesito. Soy la paciente favorita de la mayoría de las enfermeras en el piso donde normalmente me atienden. Mi equipo de atención oncológica y yo hablamos de verdad. Celebramos cuando podemos y lloramos juntos cuando tenemos que hacerlo. Pido pizza para todos en el piso en las noches ocupadas para levantar el ánimo de todos, y hago todo lo que puedo entre publicaciones de videos virales y eventos en vivo con aquellos que han llegado a confiar en mí para obtener inspiración y consejos.

Ahora puedo mirarme en el espejo. Me maquillo regularmente. Me arreglo las uñas. Hago todas las cosas que necesito para sentirme hermosa por dentro y por fuera.

El amar y a vivir con mis bolsas. Son pequeños milagros adheridos a mi cuerpo. Ahora sé cómo vestirme con ropa que me haga sentir linda. Si, vivir de esta manera significa que de vez en cuando tengo que vaciar mi bolsa de ostomía en una zanja al costado de la carretera en caso de emergencia, que así sea. Vale la pena.

Aprecio cada momento en el que no estoy en el hospital, pero también aprecio los momentos en los que lo estoy. Porque estoy viva. Y tengo un propósito que es valioso para mí y mi legado.

Amor Propio al Fin

He sufrido más trauma del que nadie debería sufrir. Yo sé eso. Sé que mi corazón se rompió desde muy joven. Sé que cometí grandes errores y lastimé a las personas que amo. Pero también sé que todo eso, todo el dolor y la angustia, *es* lo que me hizo lo suficientemente fuerte como para perseverar en mi viaje contra el cáncer.

Ahora veo todo de manera diferente. Ahora me miro de otra manera.

Amo mis errores y las formas difíciles en que he tenido que aprenderlos. Me han hecho humilde, agradecido y sabio.

Me encantan mis bolsas. Mantienen mis pies en esta tierra para bailar con mi hija, orar con mi hermana y poco a poco comenzar a sanar mi relación con mi mamá. Mis bolsas me permiten viajar a Miami para pasar tiempo con mi familia. Me han permitido organizar eventos presenciales en los que comparto mi historia completa con personas que me aman y en esos momentos y espacios, me siento tan completamente aceptada y amada, que es difícil encontrar las palabras adecuadas para describirlo.

Me dan la capacidad de concentrar mi energía en cumplir mi propósito compartiendo cada vez más de mi historia con las personas que encuentran sanación y apoyo en ella.

(Y sí, Jerrod y yo todavía estamos juntos, a pesar de que nuestro matrimonio está más roto ahora que nunca. No estoy segura de lo que nos depara el futuro, pero no voy a usar el tiempo que me queda en esta tierra para estar enojada o herido por el hombre que ignora por completo la fuerza que he necesitado y los desafíos que he soportado solo para estar aquí).

Y sobre todo, me amo a *mí misma*, por primera vez en mi vida. Acepto la tranquilidad, veo la belleza de los detalles de la vida y estoy orgullosa de ser un ejemplo de resiliencia para tantos. Es el cáncer el que me ha llevado a este punto. Sin él, no creo que hoy estuviera aquí para contar mi historia.

Y por eso siempre diré que el cáncer me ha salvado la vida.

NICOLE "COCO" ROPER

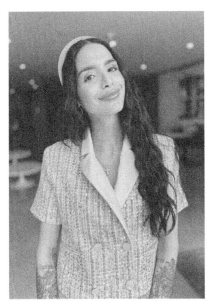

Nicole "CoCo" Roper es oradora motivacional, asesora de vida, heroína contra el cáncer y defensora de la discapacidad. Al ser dolorosamente transparente sobre su trayectoria contra el cáncer, CoCo atrae a las personas a su mundo, en línea y en persona.

Comparte todo, bueno o malo, con una comunidad de más de 100.000 seguidores en Instagram y TikTok. CoCo también habla en eventos con entradas agotadas como "Café con CoCo" y talleres motivacionales diseñados para inspirar a las personas a la felicidad.

CoCo creó marcas de moda de seis y siete cifras antes de su diagnóstico de cáncer. A pesar de una vida personal traumática, CoCo ha demostrado ser una emprendedora brillante cuya marca CoCoStrong representa la resiliencia contra todo pronóstico, tanto en EE. UU. como en Costa Rica.

CoCo inspira a otros a amarse a sí mismos y aceptar sus difíciles viajes. Su libro, Look at Me, que detalla su vida de trauma, resiliencia, amor, pérdida y propósito profundo, saldrá a la venta en febrero de 2024. Para recibir una notificación cuando se publique, visite Instagram.

Síguela en las redes sociales para conocer más sobre la historia de CoCo.

Instagram y TikTok: @IAMCOCOSTRONG

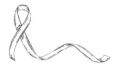

CHAPTER FIVE

CANCER CAN BE SWEET

by LaCountess R. Ingram

At first glance, the title might have made you raise an eyebrow. You might wonder, "Has she completely lost her senses?" But bear with me. Cancer can indeed be sweet, though I certainly didn't think so when I was first diagnosed.

Have you ever bought peaches, nectarines, or plums that were too hard and lacked sweetness? As a child, I recall how my grandmother would deal with unripe fruit. She'd place them in a brown paper bag, seal it, and leave it on the kitchen counter. After a few days, she'd open the bag to reveal the fruit that had become soft, sweet, and delectable.

In many ways, that's what the experience of cancer was for me. It took me—a hard and sour piece of fruit—and put me in a metaphorical brown paper bag. Over six years in that challenging space, through God's grace, I transformed. I became softer, more mature, and kinder.

Now, twenty-two years later, I'm reaching out to uplift you.

I'm here, having survived, to share my story and reassure you that you can, too. There was a time when I hesitated to talk about my cancer journey, fearing that even mentioning it would bring it back. That fear is gone now—it is time to share and inspire hope.

God spared my life so I could say to you, "You will pull through!"

In the pages ahead, you'll see how I learned to find sweetness in cancer. What you're about to read might plant a new seed in you, nourish a seed already sown, or kindle the passion you have for God. Whatever it does, I am certain that God will bless you with healing. I am merely

69

His vessel, spreading His message of love and hope. So settle in with your favorite drink, breathe deeply, and let me share my transformative journey through cancer.

The Problem

My bout with cancer was what I've come to call a "Manufacturer's Moment." Here's an analogy: my eldest son is an avid video gamer. Once, his Playstation malfunctioned. Despite his best efforts and even taking it to a repair shop, it couldn't be fixed. Their advice? Send it back to the manufacturer. So he did. Not only did Sony diagnose and repair the issue, but they upgraded his system, enhancing his gaming experience.

My point is simply: *I needed healing.*

The disease wasn't just a physical ailment; it pointed to a deeper issue. I needed to return to the "manufacturer" for diagnosis and repair. As you'll see, my journey led to more than just healing; it brought about transformation, enriching both how others perceive me and my own self-perception. For me, cancer wasn't just a disease. It was a glaring sign that there was an internal misalignment. The word "disease" itself can be broken down to "dis-ease"—an unrest or imbalance within. So, I had to question: What was causing this unrest in my physical and spiritual being?

Valid questions, wouldn't you agree?

Reflecting on my life before diagnosis, I was grappling with various situational challenges and a whirlwind of emotions. On the surface, I was navigating life as a newly divorced woman with young children. The trauma of my then-husband abandoning our kids and me for another woman, especially while I was pregnant, left me feeling unloved and like an utter failure. We were isolated on the West Coast, far from my familial support. Miraculously, with God's grace and the assistance of my biological and church families, we made it back to the East Coast. We found refuge in my mother's house, sharing the tight space with my brother. For three years, the kids and I called her living room home as I endeavored to rebuild our lives.

As for my emotional journey, it began much earlier. As a child, I felt unique; I believed I had a special gift. At times, I would see vivid and beautiful colors just by closing my eyes. Beyond these visions, I felt a deep connection to something vast and celestial, even if I couldn't quite put it into words.

A joyful and inquisitive little girl, I was always eager to engage with others and would often strike up conversations with passersby on our street. My upbringing was largely under the care of my grandmother and mother. For the first six years of my life, I can specifically remember my grandma being the primary person to care for me. Gran was a strong, little, round woman who was in her early seventies by the time I was born. She was a minister, a missionary, and one of the founding members of the Pentecostal church I grew up in. My grandma would take me to church often during the week and all day on Sunday. She would cook meals for the sick, and I'd help her deliver them; she'd call people on the telephone to pray with them, and we'd also visit the local hospital to pray for those hospitalized.

Funny fact: I feel like I learned how to read the Bible before I learned to read any other book!

We ended each day with a testimony of God's goodness. Then, she would read me a story from the Bible before I went to bed. Gran took care of me as best as she could, but in her mid-seventies, her health began to fail. She lost her eyesight and had crippling arthritis. She was not able to go up the steps anymore, so we turned the dining room into a hospital room. We wanted to honor her request to not be placed in a nursing home.

As I grew and got older, it was more apparent to me I did not have a traditional family with a mom and dad like my friends did. Over time, that childlike joy and enthusiasm began to diminish. My ability to see vivid colors was sporadic at best. My mother, although she was physically around, worked from 3 p.m. to 11 p.m. Because of her work schedule and her life struggles, she was not there for me emotionally until much later in my life. Mom and I rarely spent time together, and when I tried to talk to her, she'd tell me to shut up and leave her alone. She would yell at me and say hurtful things. I'd get beatings for no reason. She would tell me that I talked too much. She said that when I got older, I would need to find a job that involved talking because I never shut up. I was in so much pain. As a child, I can remember having pretend conversations with her in my mind.

Mom, why are you mad at me?

What did I do wrong? I know you have to work, and you are tired, but can we talk?

Can we go out and spend time together? Do you have to yell at me so much?

Wait! No, another beating, Mom!?

What did I do now? I'm sorry, Mommy. I will do better.

If I clean this, will you still be mad?

Mom, do you have to smoke that again?

As for my father, I was abandoned and rejected by him. He was from Haiti. My parents were engaged to marry, but he left before I was born. I first met him when I was six and again ten years later, at sixteen.

As a young girl, I recall thinking:

Dad, where are you? Don't you love me? What did I do wrong?

Can we just spend time together? Do you even care?

I know you have another wife and kids, but can I please be included in your family?

I need you, Daddy! I am so sorry.

I will learn to speak your native tongue and make you proud of me.

Please just come back. It is scary and lonely here.

I'd write him letters, but he never responded. His lack of response pushed down my ability to see color at all. As a result of a childhood filled with trauma and rejection, I was left to wonder if I was lovable at all.

I longed and ached for love from my parents. A hollowness inside me began somewhere between seven to nine years of age and intensified after my brother was born. I was excited to be a big sister, and I loved him. It's just that I found it hard to be truly happy. His dad came around more than my father, and even though his father would show me kindness, it was not the same. I always felt my brother was loved more because my mom had a better relationship with his father.

You could say the problem for me was deep emotional pain and distress. The emotional layers of unworthiness and feeling unlovable began to frame the way I experienced the world.

I felt very little motivation, and taking care of myself became difficult. I was critical, judgemental, and harsh with others because I was that way with myself. My voice was taken from me as a young girl, and I learned early in life how to tuck it all inside and swallow the pain. This left me frustrated because I wanted to speak, but nobody heard me or understood me. I was told I was evil and nasty and that I had a bad attitude. But no one knew the pain I was in or the fear I had.

I feared love. When I tried to love, it would end up leaving me feeling unlovable. It would hurt.

I was afraid to live and afraid to speak out for fear of judgment. I wanted to say something, but whenever I tried to articulate what was going on or how I felt, I was told to shut up and that I talked too much.

So, I swallowed what I wanted to say and suffered. I swallowed the anger. I swallowed the hurt, the pain, and the unforgiveness. I allowed fear to be a guide. I found myself doing things to be loved, accepted, and wanted. I wanted to be heard, but my attempts seemed to mute me even more. I accepted Christ into my heart as Savior around age nine, but I did that more out of fear of dying and going to hell than anything else.

As I entered adolescence, I found some relief in playing sports, but my desire to be loved caused me to look for it in places I am not proud of. I was an emotional wreck. The emotional dis-ease had started long before I got married, so I fell for the dysfunctional attention he showed me. I was broken and fragmented, and my view of love, life, and men was very distorted.

Ironically, I married someone who was just as emotionally wrecked as I was. Hurt people hurt people, and we hurt each other. Worse, we hurt our kids.

The Diagnosis

My life before the diagnosis was hurried and intense. I rushed here and there, always busy doing this and that but never really accomplishing anything. I'd start something but not complete it. I would search for love, endeavoring to fill the emptiness, but every attempt left me even more hollow.

I remember joining groups in search of love and a sense of belonging. I was an angry, bitter, frustrated, hurt, and unforgiving individual who was living in survival mode. I was going through the motions. And I was not always there for my kids. In some ways, it was a lot like how my mom had been with me, but with some differences. Nevertheless, it's safe to say that I was checked out emotionally.

It felt like a cycle I would never escape. Yet, to look at me, you would never have known my life was a wreck.

I worked hard to appear joyful and happy despite my world being framed with fear, guilt, and the feeling of unworthiness.

In March 2000, I was diagnosed with papillary carcinoma—three years after my youngest daughter's birth and two years after my divorce from their father. Things had just started to look up. I had secured a good-paying job and rented a duplex for the kids and me. We had finally moved into a place of our own. We each had our own bedroom. Things were good.

Then I noticed I was feeling tired. But as a single mom with young children, that was expected. So, I went to the doctor for my routine annual physical. My blood work was normal; however, the doctor discovered one side of my neck was slightly larger than the other. I personally had not noticed it, but she did and felt it was significant enough to have it assessed further. Thank God she did because a fine needle aspiration confirmed that I had papillary carcinoma.

Cancer?!

I went numb. *But I am only 29… And I have these beautiful kids to raise! Surely, God, you did not give me these beautiful inheritances only to take me from them! Please tell me it ain't so!*

An image flashed through my mind: I saw a coffin at the front of a church and my kids being raised by my aging mother. It was terrifying. I drove to my mother's house. She was taking a bath, but I didn't care. I stormed through the bathroom door and began to sob. My mother assured me we would get through this together and that she'd be there with me each step of the way.

I later went home to the kids. I helped them with homework, gave them dinner, and put them to bed. And once they were settled and out of earshot, I fell on my knees and cried out to the Lord, "HELP ME, LORD!"

The Healing

My experience with cancer was a six-year journey with lymph node involvement and some metastasis to my voice box. In a very real way, I deeply believe that my cancer diagnosis was a manifestation of all the negative emotions and experiences I had swallowed years before.

After being diagnosed, all the emotions I had been feeling already were exacerbated. The fear in me was really big. The anger, the unforgiveness, the hurt, pain, and anxiety all started to well up within me. I wanted relief. I did *not* want to stay stuck in this place. And Lord knows I did not want to die in this state with all these raw emotions. I needed healing, but I was afraid to talk to my heavenly Father for fear that God would treat me like my earthly father—by leaving and rejecting me. Instead, He showed me something different, and thus, my healing began with Him and our relationship.

My cancer diagnosis made me question everything. I knew something was not right and I wanted to know what it was. So I prayed to the

Lord and asked, "What's going on? What am I going to do? I want to be healed!"

I told a pastor friend all my concerns. What he replied to me changed my life—and my relationship with God—forever. He said, as a child of God, I had a right to ask Him for an understanding of the trial I am in.

"God is not intimidated by your questions, LaCountess. Ask Him!"

My friend was right. God encouraged (and continues to encourage) us all to come to Him and ask (Matthew 7:7; Isaiah 1:18). This information helped me through the cancer journey, and it guides me even until this day. My friend also instructed me to "joy read" through the first four books of the New Testament to familiarize myself with the life and ministry of Jesus Christ because every sick person who encountered Christ was healed. He told me to be open to what I would learn and receive the healing that would come. I trusted what he said, and I did as I was told.

The many lessons I learned transformed my life.

You see, Friend, the Lord showed me that a relationship with Him is a lot like my relationship with my kids. As a parent, I know when something is wrong with them. I can ask them what is wrong, and if they do not discuss it with me, they are not allowing me into their situation to help them. However, the moment they tell me what is wrong they are inviting me in so I can listen and help them.

I believe the healing began for me the moment I fell on my knees and prayed to the Lord for help. He knew what was wrong with me, but He wanted me to talk to him about it. Prayer is having a conversation with God, and it is the way we invite God into our situation.

Now, Friend, I want you to know that we can always talk to God and ask Him for a better understanding of the trial we are facing. Just *be ready for His answer*. It may not be what you are expecting, but *He will answer*.

When I asked for a better understanding of this illness, God spoke to me through a Sunday school class I took. He said to look at the issues of my heart.

Jeremiah 17:9 says, "The heart is deceitful and above all things and beyond cure. Who can understand it."

Only God knew my heart, and only He could cure and heal it, and that is what He did. He gave me a new heart.

My healing started inward, with my heart, and then proceeded outward. The more I read the Bible, the more it transformed me. I had a lot of questions (which was nothing new), and because my relationship with Christ was developing in this dark space of my life, I was getting answers while He was developing me.

To see God and learn about His vast love for me changed the trajectory of my life. You see, as a kid being raised in a strict Pentecostal church environment, I was introduced to a God of judgment, fire, and brimstone. I was taught about the anger of God but never about the love of God. I was told never to question Him, and so He scared me. But the God I learned about through this cancer journey in my twenties was loving. I discovered God had good plans for me. He had an expected future for me, and His desire was for me to receive His love and share it wherever I go.

In James 1:17, it tells me that only good and perfect things come from Him. And so I did not believe that my cancer came from Him, nor did I believe He was mad at me or that this was punishment. Instead, the Bible tells me in Jeremiah 31:3 that He loves me with an everlasting love, and He rejoices over me with singing (Zephaniah 3:17). I am the apple of His eye (Psalm 17:8). And whether you believe it or not, you too are loved.

God's desire is to know us, and He wants us to know Him! Cancer was the agent used to cultivate my relationship with Him. My cancer experience made me look more closely at the issues in my heart and draw closer to God. To look at the pain, the hurt, and the unforgiveness that encrusted my heart. Together, God and I dealt with the abandonment and rejection issues together. He showed me that even though my earthly father abandoned and rejected me, He will never leave me or forsake me (Deuteronomy 31:18; Matthew 28:20). Each encounter I had through prayer and reading His precious love letters to me, I was pushed closer to a more intimate relationship with Him. The hard edges and sharp corners of my heart began to soften in the midst of going through such a trying and arduous time. I began to see color again when I closed my eyes. And forgiveness started to flow.

My mom was with me the whole time and through that process, I began to see her differently. I forgave her, I forgave my father, I forgave my ex-husband, and I forgave all others who hurt me.

I've grown, and I am still growing. With every trial, every challenge, and every difficult space I find myself in, I know that it is there to make me better, not bitter. Each time I read about the challenges and trials faced by so many different people in the Bible, I recognize that they came through it with their faith in God growing even stronger and their relationship with God growing to new levels. Because of cancer, I was able to invite the Healer into different areas of my life where, together, we were able to expose the layers of hurt and pain so that we could recover and reclaim what had been stolen over the years—and then rebuild my life with Him as the lead carpenter.

Friend, I recognize you are in a difficult and trying space right now. I understand this is *my* testimony about *my* cancer journey; however, cancer may or may not be your agent. It could be lupus, the death of a loved one, or a financial loss. Perhaps it is the after-effects of abuse, mental illness, or divorce … I want you to know the Healer is here as you read this book to heal you. Invite Him in and allow His love to transform and soften any and every hard area in your heart. Simply say, "I invite you in, Lord. Forgive me. Help me!" With every difficult challenge that comes, there is an opportunity for you and me to grow in our faith and relationship with God, with others, and with ourselves!

Rebirth

The process of being reborn is referred to as rebirth. You could say I was reborn during my cancer journey. And Friend, I am no stranger to the term reborn because of my upbringing in the church.

At the age of nine, I remember asking Christ to forgive me and come into my heart; however, it was during my cancer journey that I discovered the truth: even though I asked God into my heart, there was still something *I* needed to uncover for myself.

There was a point in my journey when I had undergone surgery and treatment and was doing well. That was, until I went for a check-up, and they discovered it was back—this time with lymph node involvement.

I was scared all over again because I did not want to die. My kids were so young, and I wanted to be there to raise them. I was filled with anxiety. I was still trying to recover financially, and my resources were limited.

How will we eat? Will we be evicted? Will the kids' schedules be disrupted? What will the surgery and treatments be like? Will I lose my hair?

I believed with all my heart I was here on this Earth for a specific reason, but would I be able to do what I felt my calling was? As I mentioned before, cancer pushed me closer to the Lord.

So, quite naturally, I began to talk to Him: "I thought we were cool! You showed me the areas I needed to look at, and I am so blessed we did, but what is this? It's back … Do you see this?"

The ways I had previously grown closer were still there through reading the Bible and prayer; however, I began to incorporate journaling. Prayer is simply talking to God honestly and openly.

During this phase of the journey, I learned I don't have to have eloquent speech when I pray and it does not have to be long or drawn out because there were times when I was too weak to say a long drawn-out prayer. There were days when all I could muster up was, "Help me, Lord." And then there were days I had so much to say that I'd journal it and read it to God as a prayer. I'd read scripture, write it in my journal, and then write out what it meant to me. This took my understanding to a whole new level, and I started to see that God is always speaking, but because of the busyness of life, I did not always hear Him.

Now, Friend, I know you are probably thinking, "Really, LaCountess? God *spoke* to you?"

I am here to tell you, "Yes! He spoke!" He spoke to me (and continues to speak to me) through the Bible. He spoke to me through people like my pastor, He spoke to me through nature, and there was an instance He spoke to me through a billboard. I was having a tough time when I learned the cancer was back. I was scared to go through surgery again, and I did not want to go through it. The first doctor who operated on me told me the location where they saw the cancer was not in his area of expertise, so he referred me to the Hospital of the University of Pennsylvania. I began to ask the Lord about this place and whether I should get the surgery. Then, one day, as I was driving to visit a friend, I saw a billboard that said, "Penn Medicine, we see life ahead."

At that moment, I felt in my heart it was God's way of saying, "Yes, this is the place."

I was in awe of God and discovered a deeper sweetness and intimacy that amazed me because I did not realize I could go deeper into His love. I thought, "He really loves me enough to help me pick the right hospital?!"

The answer was and is: *Yes*! God loves you, and He loves me … AND he wants to be involved in every aspect of our lives. He wants us healed and doing well in every area of our lives: physically, relationally, spiritually, financially, emotionally, and mentally.

My final surgery was on February 16, 2006; however, in the final weeks before the surgery, I felt a tug at my heart and knew it was the Lord. I still was struggling with fear and unworthiness. Yes, even though I had great breakthroughs, I was still having breakdowns, but I had faith and knew that I would somehow get through it. Getting through the breakdown may not always be the way I want or envision it, but I will get through it because my greatest breakthroughs are on the other side of the breakdown.

The tug I felt at my heart was God's way of saying to me, "I see you. Let's talk."

I began to read the Bible, pray, and journal. As I went through the four gospels again, I reread about the woman with the issue of blood (Mark

5:24-34) and the man at the pool of Bethesda (John 5), and I heard the Lord say to me, "LaCountess, healing has never been an issue for me, I can do that, but what are you going to do when I heal you? Will you go back to the life you had before the diagnosis?"

Needless to say, I was at a loss for words. I wanted and needed to change because life before the cancer diagnosis was ugly, and I could not afford to go back there. So, I continued to posture my heart to receive, hear, and heal.

On February 14, 2006, while in the shower, as I felt the warm cleansing water fall on me, I heard a quiet voice say, "Daughter, you asked me to come into your heart many years ago, but you never gave me your heart. Give me your heart, LaCountess."

I stood there crying, with my hands raised in the shower, and I gave my heart to the Lord. This act of giving my heart to the Lord ushered in the greatest deliverance and healing I never thought possible. I forgave myself. I forgave myself for the past failures and mistakes I made. Through His love and grace for me, I was able to fully extend that love and grace to myself and to others.

Talk about REBIRTH!!

I was reborn in my prayer life, my vertical relationship with the Lord, and my horizontal relationships. They all became stronger. God became my filter, and I learned to love and trust through Him. Those ugly things that layered themselves over my heart, God took them and gave me a new heart that beats with His rhythm of love. And my ability to live and thrive freely was restored. The decisions I made and the relationships I attracted from that hurt and unhealed place were now made from a place of healing and wholeness.

Through God's grace, my relationship with my mother healed, and we became friends. I found my dad and reconciled with him. I was able to forgive my ex-husband, and I started to pray for him. I found myself sincerely wanting him healed and whole, too. Best of all, love found me, y'all, and I married the man of my dreams in 2014.

My Assignment

I have been asked to partner with these amazing Cancer Heroes to share my story and secrets that will combat fear and kickstart hope and healing. Dear Heart, I know this process is frightening, and fear arises. I want to support you by saying: acknowledge the fear but do not stay stuck there.

Psalm 27:1-2 says, "The LORD is my light and my salvation whom should I fear? The LORD is the strength of my life of whom shall I be afraid?"

God is here for you. Run into the sanctuary of His love and receive His love and healing.

You may be newly diagnosed, or you may have been on the cancer journey for a bit, but please do not fear and allow the love shared in this book to comfort you. Hope is an expectation, want, or desire for a certain thing to happen.

The other authors and I are here to stand with you in faith that your desire for healing will take place. The process of becoming sound and healthy again will happen. I am so grateful for this opportunity and do not take it lightly.

Friend, I prayed a lot throughout my cancer journey. If you find yourself doing the same, that is a good place to be. My prayer life was developed during this journey, and with each subsequent trial that has come, my prayer life grows stronger.

* * *

One of my prayers throughout this cancer journey went something like this:

"Lord GOD, I am scared! I want to live. I want to raise my kids. The things You have placed me here to do, great things on Earth I haven't even started to do them. Father, I know whatever you decide is a win/win for me. I want to live, and if You bring me through cancer and allow me to live (which is what

I want to do: LIVE!) I will tell people about You wherever I go. I will talk about and write about Your love and healing to whoever is willing to listen. I will proclaim your goodness wherever I go. And Lord, should You decide to take me from this Earth, I will live with You forever, so I win no matter what. Just to be clear, Lord, I want to live.

In Jesus' name, this is my prayer. Amen."

His answer came to me out of Mark 1:30-31:

"Simon's mother-in-law was lying in bed with a fever, and they told him about her at once. So he went to her, took her by the hand, and raised her up. The fever left her, and she began to serve them." God said to me, "LaCountess, you are healed to serve."

In 2 Corinthians 1:3-5, it says:

"Blessed be the God and Father of our Lord Jesus Christ, the Father of mercies and the God of all comfort. He comforts us in all our afflictions so that we may be able to comfort those who are in any kind of affliction through the comfort we ourselves receive from God. For just as the sufferings of Christ overflow to us, so also through Christ our comfort overflows."

* * *

In my journey through cancer, I got to experience firsthand the comfort and healing of the Lord, and now it's time for me to use my voice to comfort others with the comfort and love Christ overflowed to me.

My assignment is very simple: To use my voice to bring hope and healing, to pray for anyone enduring trauma, and to reignite what may have been snuffed out as a result of life's traumas that layered you up. I do this through speaking life, strength, and encouragement, which will fan the embers of greatness in you and propel you into your destiny.

When I think back on my journey through cancer, I feel like having cancer was an attack on my assignment and purpose in life. Now that I am on the other side of the journey, I see clearer now. I went through cancer for the assignment—my purpose—to come forward. I understand better now that not every trial is the consequence of wrongdoing. Sometimes, we go through it to birth something greater out of us that otherwise never would have been produced.

Cancer came to destroy but instead, it pushed me back to the Creator. The physical manifestation of cancer was the result of something deeper, and He wanted me to come to Him for proper diagnosis and treatment. He wanted me to come through it, to strengthen, encourage, and heal others. Friend, I am healed that I may serve others. God healed me and filled me with His love and light so that I may love and ignite others. My voice was given back to me to empower others, and words cannot express the excitement I feel knowing this.

So I say to you, Friend, healing is not a problem. God can heal you. The question is, what are you going to do when He does?

I want you to think back to when you were a young child; that is who I want to speak to in this moment. What beautiful gift and talent flowed effortlessly from you as a child? What was your superpower as a child before the layers of darkness attached themselves to you?

Perhaps, like me, you talked a lot. Maybe you sang all the time and had the ability to see color even when it was dark and gray. Maybe you were good at playing an instrument, or you had an artistic flair and propensity for drawing. Maybe you had an amazing ability to make people laugh or bring them comfort.

Ponder that for a moment.

Our assignment and purpose were placed in us BEFORE we were formed in our mother's womb.

Jeremiah 1:5 says, "I chose you before I formed you in the womb; I set you apart before you were born. I appointed you a prophet to the nations."

Whenever I read this, it confirms for me that God placed our assignment and purpose in us before we were born. In other words, I am a purpose named LaCountess, and you are a purpose named

_____, and everything we need to fulfill our purpose and destiny is already inside of us.

I read a quote from an unknown author that stated, "Children are lamps to be lit and not lamps to be filled."

Think about that for a moment.

It is the parent's duty to cultivate and ignite what is already within the child. Unfortunately, that does not always happen. I know that was not the case for me. The trauma and negative experiences prior to my diagnosis of cancer layered me up and sequestered the authentic me. But I am free now, healed so that I can speak to the person burdened with hurt and dysfunction. And I speak life.

Hold on, and don't give up. Be healed, Friend!

Since my last surgery in 2006, I have served in several capacities, and I will continue to serve as God leads me. I have experienced more trials, challenges, highs, and lows. That's life. I know the trials will continue as long as I live on Earth. However, it was my journey through cancer that gave me the chance to see there is a sweet opportunity to grow.

Within every trial and challenge, I gather the tools I need to weather the subsequent storms.

It was my journey through cancer that helped me grow in my relationship with the Lord, my parents, and myself. I never want to go through that again, but I am grateful that, as a result, I have reestablished healthy relationships, a healthy view of myself, healthy love, and a better awareness of what I need to do to maintain my well-being. That is sweet to me.

In 2019, my precious husband, James, suddenly passed away. It has by far been one of the toughest journeys yet. Experiencing life on Earth without him is hard, but the tools I gleaned in my cancer journey are aiding me through my grief. I know I will see James again; however, the greatest comfort is knowing God's love and comfort will get me through this season of loss as He did when I had cancer.

Friend, I do not fully understand why God chose to take James so suddenly. I simply trust Him. And, out of the pain of losing my husband, my purpose manifested—Healed to Go, LLC was born.

I am so blessed as a result of it.

I get to ignite and coach layered people who want to uncover the layers, heal, transform, and go forth in their God-given destiny. This is done through empowering conferences, corporate workshops, writing books, consulting, and teaching the empowering message of God. I coach people on how to live, thrive, and be well. It is so rewarding. More importantly, I get to fulfill the promise I made to God when I journeyed through cancer.

Friend, wherever you are in this process, God wants you to know He loves you and He is with you. Cancer can be sweet when we know Him and live in the light of His love.

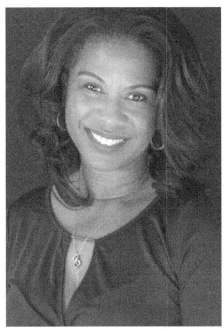

LACOUNTESS R. INGRAM

LaCountess R. Ingram is a mother, grandmother, caregiver, faith-based life and wellness coach, and a sought-after motivator and speaker. She is the founder and CEO (Chief Empowerment Officer) of Healed to Go, LLC, a conscious lifestyle experience offering transformational tools and messaging to help heal old ways of thinking and being.

LaCountess shares her journey through cancer on many platforms, where she shares the power of living well physically, spiritually, and emotionally. She is best known for her energetic, practical, and positive teaching style.

LaCountess currently serves as an associate minister and Director of Wellness at New Life Deliverance Worship Church in North Brunswick, NJ, under the leadership of Pastors Jussttinn and Cora Coleman. She is passionate about exhorting women and men to understand and unlock their value, allowing them to fulfill their God-given purpose. Visit her online at *healedtogo.com.*

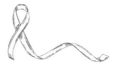

CHAPTER SIX

HEALING STORIES

by Rowena Rodriguez

D o you remember when you were a child and you heard the ice cream truck coming down the street? All of a sudden, no matter what you were doing, nothing else mattered except getting Mom to pay for that darn ice cream!

As children, the smallest things feel like the biggest things. Then, as we get older, the tasks and challenges of daily life cause us to forget what matters most: *the simple things.*

When you're faced with a life-altering situation, it can be difficult to recognize and embrace those small yet potent moments in life. All of a sudden, you notice that you have to seek them out intentionally. They no longer just appear to you.

Whether you're battling cancer yourself, supporting someone who is, or you're on a learning journey, I challenge you to live with the intention of seeking out all of those wonderful moments that make life what it is. Aim to experience every day as if you were experiencing it through the lens of a child's eye. I encourage you to experience the joy that results from rediscovering life as the miracle it is.

Hi. My name is Rowena Rodriguez. I am writing to you as a cancer survivor, a self-healing spiritual wellness ambassador, and a health advocate with a mission to inspire and transform people's lives. I have been blessed with amazing opportunities to speak on international stages, traveled to over forty countries around the world, lived in some of the coldest places on the planet, and have stared death in the face more than a few times in my life. I am a sister, a daughter, and a friend, and I'm here sharing my story with you with the hopes that inside my experience, you will find inspiration, hope, and, most importantly, the belief that anything you desire or believe can be manifested into reality.

Throughout my life, like many on this journey, I have had ups and downs, experienced heartbreak, learned great lessons from my circumstances, and witnessed many people lose their lives to many of the life-threatening experiences I've had to endure along the way.

These specific, shared moments I'm about to share with you are some of *my most potent healing stories*—the ones I feel the most compelled to share with you in this chapter.

While I am sharing my learnings along the way, I will first say that I definitely do not have all the answers when it comes to healing and overcoming obstacles.

The lessons that I have gathered have supported me in getting to the place I am today—Lupus-free. Cancer-free. And, well, free in general.

And you might be wondering, what does that even mean? To be free?

For me, it means to be at peace with your circumstances and to honor and allow whatever needs to come up in the process to come up. It means being able to be in your shadows and still remember your light. It means doing the things that bring you the greatest joy, even in the midst of tragedy, heartache, illness, and misfortune.

That's what freedom means to me.

In the next few pages, I will share stories, truths, heart-wrenching experiences, and moments that have captured my soul in ways only God and I know.

My hope is that you find comfort in my words and know, more than anything, that whatever it is you are going through (and we are ALL going through something), you are not alone. There are people just like you and me who are going through the exact circumstances or situations we have gone through. And that raises the question: *What will we then do with what we know?*

I choose to share it with the world and pray that my words touch a part of your soul in ways that help you remember your greatness, your light, and your purpose for still being here.

I'm Still Here and So Are You

I once heard the words, "Train yourself to let go of everything you fear to lose." And they resonated with me. When it comes to life, the sheer idea of potentially losing your life is one that anyone would fear. But the reality is, I am not new to having illness in my life. In fact, it's been my companion in many ways for many years. From the age of seven, in fact.

I remember it was a hot summer day, and as I stood on the diving board at our neighbor's pool, I heard our neighbor yell out, "Remember, you are only to dive!"

The challenge was that I didn't know how to dive. I knew how to do a pin drop, where you simply jump off the diving board. However, in that moment, I was left with two choices: to dive or to jump. Seems like a simple choice, right? Well, the courageous girl in me decided that I would dive without ever diving before, and I ended up hitting my head on the bottom of the pool.

That night, I started having epileptic seizures, and they would carry on for five years, beginning my journey. It was in that moment that I learned the value of life. At seven years old, it was a frightening life experience that I will never forget: being underwater, unable to breathe, seeing the surface and yet not knowing how to get back to air, feeling helpless … Yet, I somehow knew it wasn't my time yet. I remember resurfacing and seeing my mother's face. She was standing on the edge of the pool with a face no child would want to see, filled with worry and yet also, so comforting.

As they pulled me up, I thought, *I'm still here, and I'm going to be okay.*

Then, when I woke up in a hospital room after my first seizure, my mom was by my side, rubbing my forehead, and I knew everything truly would be okay.

This experience and the years that followed were difficult for my parents. They had to watch me have seizures on several occasions. I could only imagine how frightening that must have been. In many ways, this brought me closer to them. It's interesting how certain circumstances in life shape us and our relationships with others.

One day, I was in church with my parents, and the priest said something extremely disturbing. He told me that people who have seizures have a demon inside of them! *Who tells a child that?* And, of course, my mother, being the protective lioness she is, confronted the priest and had him apologize to me. Even so, I spent years believing something was wrong with me.

And then, finally, God willing, the seizures completely stopped.

Fast forward a few years: At fifteen, I was diagnosed with rheumatoid arthritis and Raynaud's disease. If you've never heard of Raynaud's, it's a condition where you lose complete circulation in your extremities. My hands, feet, tongue, and nose would get really cold and turn white as I started to warm up. Then they'd turn blue and purple as I regained circulation. It's definitely a weird sensation and one that feels so uncomfortable in the moment.

I remember being on a class ski trip during which I couldn't actually go on the slopes with my friends because I couldn't be in the cold weather. I would spend all day sitting inside the chalet while my classmates flew down the hills. During those moments, I remember feeling alone and left behind (as I assume any child would).

And as my teenage years continued to pass, 1999 would be one I would never forget.

It was summer. I had just finished high school and was waiting for university to start when, over the course of three weeks, I lost about twenty pounds off of my 110-pound body. I began finding clumps of hair on my pillow and started having extreme pain in my muscles and joints. It was one of the scariest times in my life, and yet I was still determined to go to university. So, off I went to Ottawa for my first year of school.

I shared a dorm room with a girl named Katie, my saving grace. As so many frosh students are, I was so excited to be there, excited to step into a new experience in my life. That was, until, on my second day, I couldn't move. Literally.

Katie had to help me get to the washroom. My body felt like it had been hit by a bomb. Every inch of my body was erupting with intense pain. At the same time, I felt extremely weak. I found myself close to fainting three or four times that day.

Katie took it upon herself to call my parents and told them, "Mrs. Rodriguez, there's something wrong with your daughter. You're going to need to pick her up."

I can only imagine what was running through my parents' minds as they heard those words from my roommate. Worse still must have been the dread and impatience they must have felt on the long drive they took to reach me and see what was happening.

The unknown: one of those beautiful yet terrifying things we face in life.

Five hours later, my parents arrived. My mom said I looked like I was going to die and truth be told, I felt like it.

The next few days were awful as we returned to Toronto and scheduled visits with doctors, doing our best to try to figure out what this was.

I've always said that my mom has superpowers. She has this amazing ability to know things before they happen and to figure things out.

After doing her research, she said, "I think you have lupus."

I had never even heard of this before. That unknown was frightening to me. I wasn't sure how lupus would affect the way I lived my life.

After seeing a number of doctors and no resolution, I ended up going to see my uncle, who was a GP, to see if he had any suggestions. While I was in his office, I ended up fainting and was rushed to the Toronto Western Hospital, where I was later diagnosed with systemic lupus erythematosus—an incurable illness.

While in the hospital, I shared a room with another young lady who was also diagnosed with lupus. On the third day that I was there, she passed away. That, in addition to doctors bombarding me with information about lupus, frightened me to the core.

My mind raced. *Am I going to die? Can I die from this?*

All of these thoughts ran circles in my mind as the doctor continued to reveal what this illness was and what it would mean to my reality.

And wow, was that ever a vulnerable time! My mom had to bathe me because I was so weak. She looked me in my eyes in a way that told me she felt every part of me and what I was going through. It's something I'm sure a mother would never want to experience or see, but it was also one of the most sacred experiences we have ever shared together.

As you can imagine, this was likely one of the hardest and most challenging times in my life—one that was truly unexpected in many ways. I mean, who is ever really ready for a diagnosis like this?!

But there I was, facing this incurable illness. My life felt like it stopped. I ended up having to take a year off of school after being fully diagnosed so that I could deal with the aftermath of what the disease meant to my life.

For example, I would now have to take thirteen pills a day without knowing the impact of the medicine. Medicine would be required to help me stay alive.

One of these medications was prednisone, a very strong medication that had a lot of side effects—one of which was steroid psychosis. This medication created a mess of me. Paranoia took over me. I was hallucinating and had to sleep with my parents on the floor for months. That was when and if I could sleep at all. I would have these crazy visions of massive tomatoes chasing little me.

Sounds crazy, right?

Dad would stay up all night playing cards with me. Mom never failed to be her nurturing self and never failed to search for solutions to whatever problem I might have in my daily dealings with disease.

I learned to deal with lupus. And in doing so, I learned a lot about myself.

The years that followed were filled with moments of not being able to breathe, getting shingles a number of times (thanks to a weak immune system), and ending up in a wheelchair before eventually gaining the strength to walk again—a very humbling experience.

There were some very embarrassing moments as well, like peeing myself more than a handful of times, having my boyfriend carry me to the toilet and not make it, and gosh, so many others that now, in retrospect, I can laugh at. I share all of this to say that we can always find joy in every experience we go through.

If we choose to.

Over the next few pages, I'm going to share some insights and learnings that I pray will support you on your journey. I will share some experiences that have been pivotal moments in my life, moments that have shifted who I am while teaching me profound lessons.

The Beautiful Unknown

We often want to know where the path leads before we take the first step on an unknown journey, but what I've learned along the way is that the best journeys taken aren't always planned—they are discovered, moment by moment.

My belief is that when we stay in the vibrational alignment and frequency upon which we desire to feel, instead of worrying about what it looks like, we allow all that we desire to come to fruition. The reality of our human experience may look different physically; however, the power of creation is just that…living in the vortex of creation—always open to possibility.

I've learned that choosing to feel alive and well versus the opposite, even *if* and *when* the body is physically ill and telling us otherwise, begins in the mind and flows through the body. The spirit, mind, and body become one, and the dance begins. The evolution then expands bigger, and deeper, and before we know it, we become unrecognizable to ourselves. This constant commitment to evolution relies on being committed to the expansion and growth toward being fearless despite what our physical reality is showing us.

To me, it is neither magic nor absolute. Rather, it is an attitude and deep commitment to showing up for life in spite of fear.

I once heard someone say, "When we don't trust, we live in fear."

And when we are able to surrender, this is where freedom lives.

We become limitless.

To go places where there are no guarantees, to know there are risks but take our chances anyway, when uncomfortable becomes the norm and stretches our limits, we refine our character inside of uncharted territories.

The unknown is truly a beautiful space, as uncomfortable as it sometimes can be. Unknown—herein lives the essence of God where whispers are heard, moment by moment.

Along this journey, I have witnessed my body heal in miraculous ways, and my cells regenerate themselves. Unknown pathways are forming, and in my slumber and rest, my temple continues to do what it knows to do—be whole. And while it hasn't always been perfect, this experience has guided me to see where there may be a deficit.

To know thyself and truly love oneself—this is to live in the now. This is to live.

There is always beauty found in the unknown if and when we are willing to embrace it.

Give Yourself Over

There is something so beautiful in the ability to surrender. And yet, truly trusting and surrendering feels almost impossible at times. Discomfort is the currency of our dreams and our reality.

You might be wondering what I mean by that. Well, one thing I've learned along the way is that in order to truly be present in the experience we are faced with, we must be willing to give ourselves over to the process fully in order to receive the abundance of what the experience is meant to gift us.

This lesson is what has pushed me from pain to promise. I am passionate about helping others to see themselves for *who they are* while loving themselves *just as they are*. It has challenged me to go beyond anything I thought I actually could do and has created a relentless pursuit of what's possible in life.

Anytime I've had a massive shift in my life, it has presented itself as discomfort—moments of discomfort that appear before being thrown into the unknown are (and always have been) what drives me to *live life full out*. It has led me to the ends of the earth, motivated me to climb mountains, and created healing and wholeness within. And also to face whatever challenge may come—head-on with a resilient spirit, relentless belief, and deep knowing that all is well. For me, this is the alignment of our soul and the treasure of our spirit, all unfolding in human form to remind us to KEEP GOING. To keep climbing. To lean in and move forward. And keep asking questions.

So, wherever you are on your journey, my love, this is just a reminder: you have all you need within you right now.

Your Calling

Trust me when I say, *you are chosen*. Called. Set apart. For such a time as this. Each moment that passes continues to leave breadcrumbs, clues we are called to pay attention to, knowing that "the bread of life" (manna/God) is in every single moment. Selectively chosen to help shape, guide, expand, grow, and elevate our human experience to one so much grander than we can ever fathom. And while each moment is not always pleasant, beauty can still be found there. For its essence is the light within. It's who we are. And when we hold on to this light, surrender piece by piece, bit by bit, we realize we were made for these moments.

We were made to be extraordinary, relentless, resilient human beings who do not back down when the going gets tough. Life may sometimes present tidal waves that wash over us, and our instincts may be to play small, but in reality, we are called to have the greatest life ever created. All we have to do is surrender—give ourselves over to the process of becoming who we were meant to become. Don't be afraid to trust an unknown future to a known God (or whatever you conceive Him to be). Through deep surrender, we are free. We are chosen. We are what we say we are.

The greatest message I can give to anyone who is suffering is that there is a force within us stronger than any storm, brighter than any star, deeper than any ocean … and it is utterly and entirely and only yours. Awaken it, and you will receive its power.

* * *

It was August 2020 when my life changed once again. Months before that, I had noticed some changes in how my body was feeling. Being so intuitive with my body, I could feel that my vibrational energy was shifting. I noticed inflammation that was very uncomfortable. And the discomfort was growing.

Through a lifetime of experience, I knew better than to ignore it. I had to take action.

The following week, I went to the family doctor's office, and as they examined me, it was recommended that I make an appointment with a specialist. So, I did.

A couple of weeks later, I was sitting in the hospital, and the resident doctor came in. He examined me and gave me "the look." *We all know the look.* The one we get that tells us there's so much more to it than the words coming from their mouth.

A feeling of fear came over me in that moment.

What if it was cancer?

My mind began to run through an assortment of horrible potential prognoses until I stopped myself. I remember one of the lessons that I teach to this day. And it's one that has helped me along this tumultuous journey: *There is no point in making assumptions about something I have no control over at this moment.*

I've learned that there is something so profound in being *with* whatever it is we are presented. A power I would say that lends itself to surrender. At times like that, simply having the skill to be still and to breathe is a saving grace.

It was two of the longest weeks of my life before they called me back in.

When I returned to the Princess Margaret Hospital on that fateful day, I was headed into the oncology ward.

I wondered what it was in my frequency and vibration that had called me into this space.

I immediately tried to return to my safe space—the present moment, to be IN the present moment. I was taken to a patient room. I was feeling anxious and I remember hearing the door open and a middle-aged woman walking through it. The woman told me that I was diagnosed with a very rare form of cancer, squamous cell carcinoma, and then everything after she said that was a blur …

I actually do remember most of her words, but it was as if I was in a tunnel, and everything sounded muffled.

She gave me my options and basically said that I needed to make a decision as soon as possible for fear of it growing and spreading. The options she presented were to do surgery and basically take out parts of my body in my sacral area—parts that are so sacred to me and any woman. I thought to myself: *There has to be another solution.*

As I took in all of her information, I remember walking down the steps and standing in the middle of the walkway, completely distraught.

I called my mom. No answer. Called my sister. No answer. Called my dad. No answer. Then I called my partner, who picked up the phone. As he listened to me sob on the phone, his words comforted me.

"We are going to get through this together, okay?"

And what do we do? We won.

In that moment, I knew that however it unfolded, I was taught to have the heart of a champion and that I would do whatever it took to win. The reality, though, was that I was beside myself! Even though deep down I knew this was my truth, I was terrified. As I walked toward my car, I realized that I couldn't remember where I parked.

Really?! Only thirty minutes had gone by, but I couldn't remember where I parked.

Up and down the streets of Toronto I went, unable to locate my car. Finally, I spotted a police officer and told him what had happened. He kindly took me in his car, and we drove up and down the streets, looking for my car. And then, finally, we found it. *Thank God!* I thanked the officer, got in my car, and sobbed even more. I still couldn't believe it.

As days passed, I knew I had to make a decision. So, I started picking up the phone and asking people in my community who they knew. Herbalists, homeopathic doctors, alternative medicine practitioners … You name it, I contacted it.

After about two weeks, I found a holistic doctor who ended up being in Modesto, California. What was interesting about this was that my partner, Byron, lived in California, and we had been in a long-distance love affair since March of 2020. How is it that the *one* doctor I wanted to go see was in California?

I took that as a sign from the Universe and God that this is where I was called to be.

A couple of months later, I was still in California, now researching additional treatments I believed could help me. You see, I didn't want to do conventional medicine. After so many years in treatment for lupus, I was set on doing everything naturally.

I found a clinic called Sanoviv in Mexico, and forty thousand dollars later, there I was.

The center was beautiful, right off the coast of Baja, Mexico. All of the food was organic and plant-based, and every treatment was intentionally created with the patient in mind.

I tried Bio-Frequency, Hyperbaric Oxygen Chambers, High Doses of Vitamin C and other supplements, Ozone Blood Irradiation, Hypothermia … If it was there, I did it. Unfortunately, even with all of these different modalities, the doctor still suggested surgery. So, I needed a plan.

I remember praying on my knees, asking God for guidance and clarity. And well, that guidance led me to Irvine, California, where I would spend the next year getting treatment at the Center for New Medicine.

Many of the treatments mirrored what I had done in Mexico, so it seemed like the right thing to do until one day when I wasn't feeling well. I was doing my Vitamin C drip and noticed my temperature was rising. The nurse ended up coming to see me and suggested I call the doctor. After a long drive home, my fever wasn't going down so he suggested I go to the hospital. I did as I was told and ended up in the hospital, where they diagnosed me with sepsis—which is life-threatening.

I thought to myself, *Are you serious? First, a cancer diagnosis, then this?*

I couldn't believe it. But there I was, being put on high doses of antibiotics and stuck in the hospital yet again.

In all honesty, though, it ended up being a huge blessing. And here's why.

The doctor suggested that I do a CT Scan. He said that since I was already there, perhaps it would make sense to just check to make sure the cancer hadn't spread anywhere else. Little did I know this would end up dramatically changing the trajectory of my journey.

I later found out that even with all of the treatment I was getting at the Center for New Medicine, cancer had spread to my lymph nodes, pelvis, and abdomen. I couldn't believe it.

I remembered thinking, *How was it that I've been doing everything I should be doing—going to treatment, eating plant-based foods, doing cleanses, exercising when I had energy—and yet still, my cancer has spread?*

Following this news, I knew I had to do something drastic.

After much contemplation and many conversations, both my family and I made the decision that it was time to seek out conventional doctors.

And this would begin yet another journey of discovery.

After going to see at least six different doctors, of which most told me they couldn't do anything to help me, I finally came across UCLA. Two girlfriends of mine, Ericka and Anne, both called the same doctor to try to get me into an already full schedule. And I'm so glad they did. I got the appointment.

I walked through yet another set of oncology doors, set on expressing my concern and resistance to taking anything conventional, and to my surprise, the doctor was understanding and compassionate. She said surgery wasn't an option because the tumor sat too close to my urethra and could impact my ability to urinate. I thought, *Great Start!*

They then suggested seven rounds of chemotherapy, twenty-six rounds of radiation, and a very intense form of radiation—brachytherapy—where I would need to do seven procedures in three days. Which I did. That was a journey in and of itself.

The aftermath was worse, though, as I fought through the side effects of the radiation. The pain I had to experience was excruciating and an experience I wouldn't wish on anyone.

Days were filled with laying down for most of the day, having to wear diapers, getting help with showering myself and going to the washroom, using a walker and cane to support me, and not having any appetite to eat.

As months passed, the pain, discomfort, and other side effects subsided gradually, and I gained a deep appreciation for being able to walk on my own and do all of the things I had taken for granted before.

Excerpt from Day One of Treatment

One of my favorite passages in the Bible is Proverbs 31:25: "She is clothed in strength and dignity, and she laughs without fear of the future."

So here I was: December 1—treatment day one.

To step out in faith is to go forward while believing in that which is unseen. It is to walk firmly rooted and grounded in the unknown. It's about following God's will in full obedience, even when and if I don't know what my next steps will be.

Some days, I get this *nudge* or a feeling in the pit of my stomach calling me to keep going and to *let go* and *trust*. It's that deep surrender that pushes me to allow the *unfolding* to take place. There's been so much resistance within me when it came to making this decision to step forward on this path. So many voices and opinions that I've taken into account and getting ever present to God's voice—my voice.

Each day before our feet touch the ground, we present ourselves to the almighty power of God, read a passage from Jesus Calling, and give thanks for all that is—knowing on the other side of this, there is a beautiful miracle on the way and it reminds us we are not alone. And *this*, I firmly believe.

Be Willing to Be Uncomfortable

I remember it as if it was yesterday. I had just secured a contract with the Government of Nunavut in the Arctic, a place many would like to visit yet a place many will never visit because, I mean, out of all of the places one could go, how many people would say, "Yes, I'll move to the Arctic!"

And yet, there I was, living in the North, with polar bears, the tundra, no trees, twenty-four-hour darkness, and twenty-four-hour sunlight. Now, I will say that the above example I gave in regards to the ice cream truck, well, that's who I've always been. I'm someone who is emphatically fascinated by places that other people wouldn't dare to live and experiences that many would never do. I am constantly in a state of discovery. Whether it was living with polar bears, doing mission trips in Siberia, visiting orphanages in Indonesia (and Africa and Indonesia), or climbing the second highest mountain in a Rinjani, when given the invitation to live life fully, I will always take the opportunity to climb that mountain. It was such a pivotal time in my life.

I had just ended a relationship and needed a reset. So at 3 a.m. one morning, after watching *Eat, Pray, Love*, I ended up booking a trip to Bali. It was a place I'd always wanted to visit with the intention of healing my heart. So, the next day, I went to the CEO's office of the place where I worked at the time and basically said, "I need some time." And I was willing to deal with whatever repercussions were given to me. I knew there was a possibility that I might lose my job; however, in that moment, I was more important than anything—or any job, for that matter.

And my employer looked at me and said, "Take whatever time you need." I guess it helps that this particular consulting job was one that was created for me.

So, off I went to Bali. Packed my things with the intention of healing, laying out on the beach, and sipping fresh coconut juice. I hadn't planned it, so I ended up booking a place called the Bali Entrepreneurs Resort for three days and figured I would just figure it out when I got there.

At the time, I was still taking thirteen pills a day for lupus, and something inside of me told me that this trip wasn't just going to heal my heart. It was also going to heal my body.

I decided that I was going to stop taking all of my medication—something that I don't suggest anyone do without a physician's guidance. It was what I wanted to do.

The next morning, I woke up to the sound of birds chirping in my ear. I walked down to the common area where many folks were having their breakfast. As I waited for my fresh coconut and fruit, I noticed a gentleman sitting near me looking at maps. I asked him where he was going.

"I'm going to climb the second highest mountain in all of Indonesia, standing 3726 m. You should come!" he said.

I laughed and said, "You know, I've always had it on my bucket list; however, I'm here to heal, sip on fresh coconut juice, and hang out on the beach."

We both shared a laugh, and I walked back to my room. Then, I spent the day discovering different parts of Bali, enjoying some time by the pool, and having a great meal. That night, I lay in bed looking up at the ceiling fan as it turned and turned, breathing fresh air across my body, and thought, "Why wouldn't I go? I mean, I'm here."

The next morning, I jumped out of bed and ran to the common area and saw the man about to leave. And I excitedly said to him, "I'm going to come!"

He responded with, "You are? Okay, let's go!"

Now you have to understand that I didn't have any gear with me. My whole suitcase was filled with bikinis and sundresses. Literally.

I have always been someone who will figure it out. No matter what the situation is. So I did. I found an outfitter, rented a backpack, borrowed a jacket, packed whatever warm clothes I had (which was literally just a few long-sleeved shirts), wore my three-year-old Puma shoes, and off I went.

Now, let me put this into context for you: I've never climbed a mountain before. However, you and I both know that when it comes to being a thriver and survivor, being relentless is top on the list. So, off I went into the unknown.

It would be a three-and-a-half-day trek, and little did I know what that was going to look like. I ended up getting sick during the climb, had to eat charcoal to settle my stomach, and *Thank God* for the Sherpas we had with us, or I wouldn't have survived it. Bless their souls.

The third day was probably the hardest for me. I was about an hour from the summit, and my body felt like it was about to give up. My team members ahead of me kept moving on and I told them to go ahead and leave me there. My body felt like it had enough.

I slumped down on the side of the mountain and took a deep breath. I closed my eyes and asked God to help me. And all I heard was *Rise. You need to rise up into your purpose. Rise.*

As I opened my eyes, I looked over the beautiful landscape that laid out before me and I knew I had to finish. So, with everything in my body, I put one foot in front of the next. It was a volcanic mountain, so tiny little black rocks seeped into my shoes, making them heavier and heavier with every step. I kept looking up and continued to slowly make my way up. These next few moments reminded me how, often in life, we may take one step forward and a few steps back, or in some instances we take one step forward and then have to start all over again.

The moment I got to the summit, my team was cheering me on. As I sat on the top of that mountain, all I could do was cry. I realized that every single step that got me to the top was years of healing from trauma being released from my body.

My relationship. Abuse. Sickness. All released from my body.

In that moment, I knew I was free from lupus. I cried and cried. I thanked God. I felt such deep gratitude that I had made it to the top. Here I was, having never climbed a mountain before, with no gear, and I made it. I. Made. It.

It brought back so many memories of me in a wheelchair and having to learn how to walk again, and *I did it!*

I share this story with you only because on this cancer journey, we are all going to take one step backward before having to start all over again. And yet, we will need to keep going, to keep moving forward—no matter what obstacles or hurdles we may have to face.

There are moments in which we can't see the summit. And it's in these moments that we must pull from every part of our being and say, "I'm here to win."

It is no coincidence that you're reading this right now and that you're *present* to what I am sharing. You may in fact be in this exact place, feeling like giving up, unsure of the future.

I'm here to tell you: *You are here for a reason, so lace up (even if you only have your three-year-old Puma shoes) and keep going.* The view from the top of the mountain, I promise, will be so worth it.

You got this. *We* got this.

What Do You Need, Darling?

"Even though she doesn't have all the answers, she knows the answers live within. Sometimes, all that's required is a call to pause, observe, and be present. Those who are in true alignment will always stand in that same spirit as they, too, shine their light. She observes the signs. She trusts her instincts. And she knows that there is nothing worth more than her peace."

As a lioness, I am clear that I must know how to survive in the jungle. Part of that process requires a stillness—where we must ask ourselves what it is that we need.

When was the last time you wrapped your arms around yourself and asked, "What do you need, darling?"

So often, we forget to connect with our heart space and truly lean into what it is we need. And yet, it is the most important thing we can ask ourselves. This morning, as I woke up and asked myself this very question, in this still moment, all I heard was *"PEACE."*

* * *

Going through a journey like cancer, we often experience moments of frustration. We wonder why this is all happening. It can be overwhelming, but if we do not spend this time truly connecting with our spirit, it's a journey that can overwhelm us.

I know for me, I started questioning myself, asking if *I* had created this. I mean, I come from a space where I know that our minds are extremely powerful and that thoughts can become very real things. These thoughts can spiral out of control and, at times, have us falling into a victim mentality.

In those triggering moments of our human condition, I believe we must nourish our soul, check in, and pull from God and from the Source energy that breathes life into our spirit. It is this spirit that calls us forth to selectively choose to be the warriors within. And there is nothing, nothing worth more than our peace of mind.

What I've learned through this process is the importance of protecting the gifts we were given despite what is happening in our internal world. Water those gifts as if they were fertile soil beneath the soles of our feet. Then, watch them grow. That one seed of belief can flourish into a beautiful space of *surrender* and allow us to trust the process.

And if nothing else, that power that lives deep within can break through anything that is not in alignment with what is intended for us. What is meant for us is so much greater and grander than we could ever fathom.

We must simply claim it and be the warrior we were *called to be*.

So next time you feel rushed or overwhelmed, take a moment to put your arms around yourself and ask, *What do you need, darling?*

Find Joy in Every Moment

On the days when it feels like the world is against you, and you might need this reminder: I want you to know *I've got your back.*

I want to remind you that you were chosen—chosen by the highest God, delicately and purposefully—and that you were created for a plan greater than we can ever imagine.

But how do you find *joy in every moment* of this type of journey?

Is it actually possible?

And my answer is yes. Every. Single. Day. We always have a chance and a choice. A chance because, well, if you are reading this, you have received a new day to be alive. And we have a choice because, well, if you are reading this, we get to choose how we show up on a day-to-day basis.

* * *

I know that sometimes, I let my emotions get the best of me. At times, I'm very intentional. I return to stillness and reflect on everything I am so grateful for, knowing that each moment is a blessing. My mission is always to redefine the face of illness. I want people who are up against a disease or challenge to be able to be free.

But here is the question: Can we actually feel joy in every moment?

My answer is yes! Of course, we can.

I believe it all starts with gratitude. We should never stop reminding ourselves of every great thing we have been given in our lives. And on days when you might need a reminder, I want you to know *I got you.*

I find that if I keep my focus on what I'm grateful for, I can lean into what it feels like to reflect on what I'm thankful for. And for me, that means reflecting on that feeling of joy.

I know there will be times when you wonder what this journey is meant to teach you. In these moments, I invite you to embrace it *all*. Just as it is. Awaken the light within and feel the presence of life's majestic beauty, darling. *Be in it.*

Access to joy, regardless of what you might be going through, is possible.

Breathe it in. All of it.

Breathe in the joyful resilience. Exhale the negativity.

And while at times we may stand in this unknown space, never lose sight of the light you carry within you.

Challenges arrive in our lives to stretch us and help us grow, refining our characters and sharpening our ability to discern where we are called to put our focus and energy.

That *discomfort*, that uncomfortable feeling of peeling off the layers—and even truths—we are meant to see.

So **take it all in** and remain steadfast and relentless in your life's pursuit of joy.

And no matter what, remember what you have chosen: life. And because of that, this is your golden ticket to co-create with God to live an inspired life. You are exactly where you are meant to be. It is called joyful abundance, and it's yours for the taking!

Remember My Love

Remember, my love, you are water, so cry, cleanse, flow, and let it go.

Remember, my love, you are fire, so burn, tame, adapt, and ignite newly each day.

Remember, my love, you are air, so breathe, observe, focus, and decide powerfully who you want to be, moment by moment.

Remember, my love, that you are earth, so ground yourself in the unknown, build, produce, inspire, center, and give.

Remember, my love, that you are Spirit, so connect, go inward, listen, and be in the knowing that all you need is within you. Be still and be with that whisper guiding you along the way.

Remember, my love, that some days may stretch and expand you in moments; these are all beautiful lessons meant to make our experiences in life so much fuller.

So lean into the unknown. Bask in the beauty of the dance. Open your heart to endless possibilities and miracles. Trust me; they are coming. In fact, they have already arrived, and they are within you. Remember, my love …

* * *

This was a piece I wrote when I was waiting to receive my results from a PET scan in May. I remember that day so vividly. I sat in the doctor's office after a routine appointment, awaiting the results. As we sat there anticipating the doctor's entry, she came in and said, "I'm so sorry, but I don't have your results yet."

We ended up leaving feeling anxious, thinking about what the results might be. I knew that it wouldn't help me to worry, so I took a deep breath and let it go.

As soon as we got home, we received a call: "Rowena, I just got the results back, and you had NED!"

I responded, "What is NED?"

She explained, "It stands for *no evidence of disease.*"

In that moment, I didn't know if I should scream, cry, laugh, or smile.

I was so taken aback … everything I had done, everything that had gotten me to this point … the treatment had worked! It was truly one of the happiest moments of my life.

I beat cancer! So, remember, my love, trust that the Universe is always conspiring in our favor; we have only to believe.

Be All There

There are times in life that capture our very essence when every part of us is swept away in that very moment.

It was 2019, and I was in Haiti visiting the Help Heal Humanity School, doing feeding programs for some of the most vulnerable children in Haiti. One day, we were asked to go to the Mother Teresa Home for the Dying. A hospital where women were sent who were struck with various illnesses. Each woman had a bracelet on their left wrist, which represented where they were on their death journey. Yellow represented that they had just been diagnosed with an ailment, red represented that they were further along in their disease, and black represented that they were days or hours away from death. It was a humbling experience. As I walked into the room, my spirit was drawn to a woman who was lying in bed in the corner. There was no one around her, and something inside of me called me to her. As I slowly made my way over, the other women looked at me as if to say I shouldn't go to her. However, everything in me told me to go. As I put on my protective gear, gloves, and mask, I inched my way closer to her only to see lesions on her legs, her skeletal body, and her lifeless being. I found out that she was dying from HIV, tuberculosis, and leprosy.

As I made my way to her bed, I could tell she was filled with sadness. I stood at the foot of her bed and felt called to lay down beside her. As I put my arms around her, I remember laying down with her and saying, "I love you" over and over again as I looked deeply into her eyes. In that moment, what I knew was that love doesn't need language. It is a language in itself. After hours of being with her, I remember leaving the hospital thinking that if, for one moment, she knew she was loved, seen, and acknowledged, then I had done the right thing. I found out a few weeks later that she had passed away just days after I was there with her. It made me think to myself, if I hadn't been all there, I would have missed one of the most life-changing experiences of my life.

Oftentimes in life, we can get so fixated on what we need to do, moving through life so fast and it doesn't lend itself to us being fully present. This great lesson has reminded me that every experience we are given is an opportunity for us to be all there. To be fully engaged and present when we are speaking to someone. To be all there when we are taking on a task or job. To give ourselves over to the present moment is truly being in the gift of life.

You Are Limitless

Every champion was once a contender who refused to give up. They are people who live and breathe with heart, people who acknowledge that the opinions of others do not determine one's destiny. You do. We do. I do. Never underestimate the heart of a champion whose mind has already decided they have won.

We win. It's a saying that my partner and I often share with one another whenever we are faced with difficult moments in life. In the wild unknowns, how beautiful is it to be witness to the art of surrender and to be present to the courage it takes to lean into one's truth? How beautiful is it to remain steadfast and hold that relentless belief in the beauty the unknown carries with it? As we continue to live in a space of curiosity, humility, and grace, welcome the ever-unfolding of life and the generosity of time.

We arrive into this world as energy, the most beautiful miracle, and much like the stars, wind, and ocean, we breathe life into that which is. We release the need to control and surrender to a rhythm that expands the spirit and awakens the soul. And as we release, we flow into a deeper space of who we truly are. This is where freedom lives. When we surrender to the deep yearnings within, we can open our hearts as we expand and tap into our inner wisdom, knowing that our inner compass knows the way.

Unwavering faith is to be sure, steady, steadfast, resolute, firm, and unshakable.

Being diagnosed with cancer tests our character, our faith, our spirit, our mind, and our heart. When we know who we are and we know where we come from, our belief is stronger than any doubt or fear that may show up; we then have access to peace that no person, place, or thing can offer. For it resides within. It lives in our spirit and the deep knowing of who our God is.

Every second of every minute of every hour, the world we live in is constantly changing. Our lives are filled with the excitement of the unknown, and the ultimate questions are:

How will we respond to the uniqueness of our journey and who will we be as a result?

Wouldn't you agree that both victories and hardships gift us with the most amazing blessings in life?

We can't predict the future, and oftentimes, things happen in our lives that may push us into a space of beautiful discomfort; however, what we learn along the way is that it's these moments that define who we truly are.

And what I want you to know is that as much as it may not feel like it at times, **you are limitless beyond measure**.

So, I thought I would leave you with seven things that I've realized on my healing journey that have helped me to embrace this experience we call life.

Start with God, or whomever you conceive Him to be. Each morning before my feet touch the ground, I begin with prayer and thanksgiving. Gratitude for that which is seen and unseen, for every part of my body, for opening my eyes to another day, and for feeling my heart beat against my chest. For every blessing I've been given and all that is to come. How you start your day will dictate the rest of your day.

If you dig deep into the unknown, you are bound to find a treasure. So open your arms and embrace all that is unknown. Doing so is sure to bless you with unexpected gifts.

Embracing the unknown prepares you for the worst, the best, and beyond. So trust the process.

Learning to accept and allow this is the key to surrender. We all have an Inner Compass that calls us to listen. In that silent surrender is where the magic and miracles live.

Show up as your best. You may not have control over what happens to you, but you do have control over how you show up. Understand where you are, then move into massive action toward your vision, goals, and dreams. When we show up as our best, we become fearless of the unknowns in life. This supports us in being present every moment as we breathe life into ourselves.

Humility and character ignite and illuminate who you are. Be willing to learn and hear things that you may not agree or align with. This gentle and compassionate way of being creates within us a flow and energy that exudes a beautiful and sweet posture that opens us to new ways of being.

Be willing to forgive. Forgiveness is a big one. And it begins with us. It begins with acknowledging and accepting that which is. And when we are able to forgive ourselves, we are then able to forgive others. Forgiveness is so much more than saying "I'm sorry" or releasing guilt or resentment. It is truly one of the most beautiful gifts we can give to ourselves.

* * *

My hope is that through these words, you find comfort, hope, and something that inspires you to remember that you are not your illness or circumstance.

In you, I see a beautiful light that this world needs to see. And as you continue onward, know that every single experience was meant to teach us lessons that we may not have otherwise learned without that experience.

And perhaps, all that I am attempting to ask you is to say *"thank you."*

Thank you for this experience that continues to grow and elevate who I am.

Thank you for all of the unknowns that continue to expand my heart space and connect me with who I am.

Thank you to the amazing people that have graced me during this time.

And then maybe, just maybe, it's time to put your arms around your beautiful being and temple and ask, "Darling, what is it that you need?"

Keep going. Keep growing. And know that I am rooting for you. You were chosen to be here, so wherever you are in your journey, take this time to treasure and honor yourself.

One day at a time. One moment at a time.

We got this.

All my love,
Rowena

* * *

P.S. Just two weeks ago, I found out that the cancer has come back. I share this with you because no matter what may happen, the journey never truly ends. And I don't mean the cancer journey. I mean all of this—the journey, beauty, and dance of life. As we learn how to dance with the beauty of life, every aspect of it, we soon learn that every moment is here to teach us a lesson we may not have learned without it. This is not over. In fact, it's just the beginning.

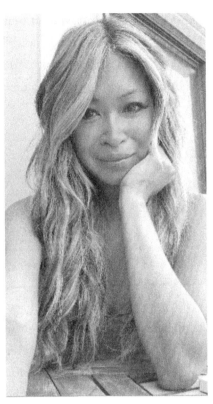

ROWENA RODRIGUEZ

Rowena Rodriguez is an international speaker, Self Healing Spiritual Wellness Navigator, and health advocate with a mission to inspire and transform people's lives. With over 20+ years of health promotion, stakeholder, and community engagement experience, her passion for community, service and authentic connections is what drives her. She believes that when we are in the service of others, we heal, miracles occur and this becomes the birthplace of possibilities.

For her, it is the legacy that matters and the possibility for each one of us to make the greatest impact we can in this world and in our lifetime. A constant theme in her world is the belief that "when we heal ourselves, we heal the world."

Website: *rowenarodriguez.ca*

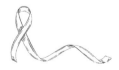

CHAPTER SEVEN

AWARENESS FROM CANCER

by Shirley Gaudon

In January 2020, at forty-two years of age, I was an emotional and physical wreck, and I didn't understand why.

Suddenly, I began gaining weight despite not eating excessively. Struggling to stay awake, I'd crash into bed immediately upon returning home, only to battle drowsiness by 9 a.m. the following day. By each workday's end, exhaustion drove me to tears. Within three weeks, rapid weight gain made my clothing from one week unfit for the next.

During one fateful shower, I discovered an odd lump in my right breast. The sheer shock held me paralyzed, making that shower feel interminably long. My fear escalated, and so I urgently contacted my doctor. Within a day, tests revealed I had hypothyroidism. Immediate medication addressed the sleep and weight concerns. However, a subsequent ultrasound identified a malignant tumor, leaving me reeling with disbelief and asking, "How did I get here?"

Eighteen years into my tumultuous marriage—characterized by deceit and excessive alcohol—my life was filled with stress, including work stress. My husband and I, both from the restaurant sector, believed in working and partying hard. The early days felt like an unending celebration. We wed after he finally proposed, despite his previous aversion to marriage—a red flag I'd foolishly challenged. Over time, I've learned to heed people's self-revelations and behaviors.

Navigating two toxic environments simultaneously was my reality, clearer in retrospect. Dysfunction in one life area often seeps into others.

From our wedding's onset, I felt deep regret, but my strict Catholic upbringing urged me forward. In both of my marriages, I overlooked early warning signs and compromised my identity. Never having witnessed a healthy relationship, even between my parents, my understanding was skewed. My father's domineering behavior left its mark, influencing my future relationships.

Pregnancy followed shortly after the wedding, leading to a devastating miscarriage. Miscarriages, a taboo in the 1980s, remained undiscussed. Yet, soon after, I was blessed with my son.

Although many believe they're prepared for marital and parental roles, reality often differs. Despite some wise decisions like buying a house, our finances were shaky. My unplanned early maternity leave left us without my income for half a year. These financial troubles were precursors to numerous challenges during our two-decade union.

With my husband working late nights, I largely parented solo, deeming myself a "married, single parent." My health complications added strain, making me increasingly reliant on my supportive mother-in-law. But the void in my marriage persisted. Over time, our relationship's deficiencies became glaringly evident.

My past had predisposed me to such a relationship. My parents' lack of constructive communication was primarily aggressive, dominated by my father. My mother's evident loneliness, seeking mere acknowledgment from my father, often resulted in familial turmoil.

Such a background made me susceptible to subsuming my identity in relationships, a trend still visible in many modern families.

Work wasn't a reprieve either. My job was steeped in a toxic culture, with coworkers at odds, leading to one particularly disturbing incident during a Montreal business meeting. Changing my job role within the same company wasn't the solution I'd hoped for.

Research has linked stress to various health issues. My tumor, attributed to heightened estrogen levels, was diagnosed only post-surgery when I underwent a biopsy after having three lymph nodes removed.

This ordeal taught me about the body's cortisol production in response to stress, which subsequently disrupts estrogen balance.

Research from the Canadian Cancer Society indicates that stress weakens our immune system. This system defends our body against infections and diseases such as cancer, thyroid malfunction, heart disease, and arthritis, among others. Stress can alter the levels of certain hormones in the body, which can heighten the risk of developing cancer. Additionally, stress may lead to unhealthy behaviors like overeating, smoking, and heavy drinking, all of which can also increase cancer risk.

Receiving the news that I had breast cancer, not knowing what type it was until I was on the operating table (and being uncertain about how far it had spread) felt like a looming death sentence. On the surface, I portrayed a strong, "no-nonsense woman" demeanor, exuding confidence that I would conquer this challenge, aiming to reassure my family. Yet, I often question if that was the right approach. Would being open about my fear and anxiety have fostered genuine conversations, allowing us all to voice our concerns and possibly find mutual support? Instead, I felt isolated, as if I had to navigate this ordeal solo. My husband, unsure of how to process the situation, became distant.

Did my apparent strength give them hope? Or did they harbor concerns about the possibility of the treatments failing?

The truth remains elusive. I later discovered that during this time, my son had confided in a friend whose mother was undergoing a similar battle, albeit with graver consequences.

I opted for the aggressive chemotherapy and radiation plan recommended by the doctors, receiving support from my family. During the nine-month recovery at home, I underwent therapy, losing my hair—a common side effect. While my husband accompanied me to some of the chemo sessions and my son joined me a few times, I faced radiation alone. Alone with my thoughts, I pondered my future, and it did not include my husband. This was my clarion call to reality. For so long, I had been numbly drifting through life. Despite the overwhelming emotions of weariness, loneliness, and unhappiness, I had become resigned to this existence. My husband's alcoholism had driven a wedge between us, and we barely spoke except for brief conversations about meals. Our meals were marked by my silence as my husband and son chatted. Intimacy had evaporated, yet we continued to share a bed. Among his numerous flaws, his tendency to lie through omission grated on me the most. Our marriage felt like a constant stream of hidden dramas, and I bore the weight of unraveling them. Love, trust, and respect had vanished, prompting me to strategize my exit.

Mimicking his father's approach, my husband provided me with an allowance for household expenses. I was in the dark about his earnings. Before my illness, I had begun saving for my own future. My goal was to amass enough to exit the marriage with my son, who had aspirations for college. I, too, hoped to leave my job and return to school, a plan I knew would take years.

This was the juncture where I truly began to reflect on my life. It was as if I had been awakened. Yet it would be years before I could truly confront and understand myself.

A recent chat with my son revealed his anger during that period. He struggled to understand my prolonged absence from work, accusing me of concealing my illness. In truth, I don't recall withholding any information. But I remember him seeking solace outside home, participating in school plays and other activities to escape the tension between his father and me. Thankfully, he found his path to healing in his late teens and early 20s, joining an Ashram program in British Columbia, which proved transformative.

I'm convinced I had informed my son about my condition since my surgery followed a month after the initial diagnosis. My reluctance to distress him was because I was unsure about the severity of the situation until the lump and lymph nodes were removed and analyzed. Only then can the true nature of the tumor, its spread, and the appropriate surgical intervention be determined. Thankfully, twenty-two years on, technological advancements have significantly improved our understanding and treatment of cancer.

Reflecting on that period, I was undoubtedly numb and consumed by fear. I convinced myself that feigning strength and building emotional barriers would carry me through. Admitting vulnerability felt like a sign of weakness. This facade deprived my family of the chance to support and comfort me—a decision I now recognize as not being mine to make. I believed that if I downplayed the gravity of my condition, it would alleviate their worries.

In retrospect, our collective journey missed an opportunity for shared healing. I remained unaware of my family's innermost feelings and whether they truly believed I would recover. While I'm uncertain if my veneer of resilience inspired them, it undeniably propelled me to confront the menace that is cancer head-on.

Subsequently, I resumed work briefly. However, it became evident that my employer was reluctant about my return. My prolonged absence due to treatments placed me in an awkward predicament between the insurance company's insistence on my return and my employer's hesitance, even implying I needn't hurry back. Upon my return, I was shunted into a new role. Merely six months later, I was dismissed without a stated cause. Their offer of assistance in job-hunting and a peculiar proposal for a farewell party—which I declined—left me bemused. The narrative provided to the staff was that I had resigned. Though they failed to find me a job, they liberated me from their manipulative grasp.

That's when I set my plan in motion. I secured a position in Human Resources as a recruiter, a role I genuinely cherished. Financial constraints tethered me to my marriage, as my son was still in high school. So, I made the decision to save more and return to school. At forty-two, I enrolled in a part-time, three-year Human Resources Management program. To my surprise, I developed a passion for learning. My earlier education was marred by stress and harsh discipline, as corporal punishment was then permissible, making my academic journey tumultuous.

Another pivotal choice was to quit drinking. I embraced sobriety for five years. Eventually, I parted ways with my husband with one year left in my course and received my certification the following year. Concurrently, I ventured into dating, which unfortunately led to a tumultuous on-again, off-again relationship. My son then relocated to British Columbia, and I experienced a prolonged period of solitude. Unaware of any resources for spiritual and emotional healing, a transformative turning point came in 2013 when I encountered Landmark Education. The remarkable women I met exuded love, joy, and prosperity, prompting me to emulate their lives. I subsequently aligned myself with a charity aiding women facing adversity, where I felt inspired to become a coach.

Today, I am a certified Grief Coach and Trauma-Informed Coach, helming my own coaching venture. I've also introduced the "Power Within Workshop," a platform empowering women to cultivate self-love, recognize their worth, and define boundaries.

I wholeheartedly champion the belief that "Everything Starts with You."

SHIRLEY GAUDON

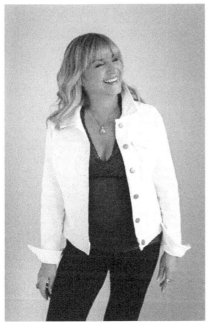

Shirley Gaudon is a Trauma-Informed Life Coach, speaker, author, and mother.

As a certified coach, Shirley focuses on helping people become more self-aware and powerful in their lives. Working through unresolved trauma allows for the creation of new roadmaps to avenues for healing and growth.

A survivor of both cancer and domestic abuse (generational trauma), Shirley designed The Power Within program. This initiative equips those seeking peace with tools to foster self-care, embrace self-love, and recognize their inherent value. It guides them on a transformative journey to rebuild, reinvent, and rejuvenate their lives. The Power Within program has been added to McMaster University Continuing Education 2023 fall semester.

With over 25 years of experience in human resources, Shirley has had the privilege of interacting with individuals across various business echelons. Her expertise has been instrumental in helping them carve successful career paths and emerge as triumphant leaders in both professional and personal spheres. Visit her online at *shirleygaudoncoaching.com*

SHIRLEY GAUDON

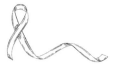

CHAPTER EIGHT

POWER OF PRAYER

by Niki Papaioannou

Before the Diagnosis

Y ou've got nothing to worry about, Niki," said the doctor at Toronto's Sunnybrook Hospital after examining the golf-ball-sized growth in my neck. It was the Fall of 2013, and it felt like the perfect time to book a trip to New York City with my good friend Maria from Cyprus to celebrate life and being alive!

Throughout the weekend, absolutely everything was going our way. So much so that each time something great would happen, Maria and I would say, "Of course!" and laugh. It became a running joke throughout the entire weekend.

On the flight home to Toronto, we even boarded the wrong plane and almost ended up in Colorado. Luckily, a flight attendant realized the error and promptly got us to the correct Toronto gate. *Of course!* What were the odds that our two specific seats on the wrong flight were open and available to us? That was just one of many things that weekend that reminded us how funny life can be. We appreciated so many moments in those three days.

Thinking only positive thoughts is easier said than done. It's especially difficult when you find yourself in a toxic workplace with a boss who seems to take great pleasure in torturing his employees. For ten years, I had a really stressful job. I was a marketing director in a very male-dominated environment. There was rarely another woman in sight. It felt almost unnatural. Even though women and men are both capable of excellent work, I don't think having one woman working in an environment made up entirely of men is conducive to success. And it certainly didn't lower the level of stress.

For three years after the Sunnybrook doctor told me the lump was nothing to worry about, I noticed that every time my stress levels would peak at work, my neck would hurt. And by January 2016, I was always aware of the lump in my throat, and it was to a point where it was visibly protruding from my neck. I was extremely worried, and I began losing weight. Yet I didn't address it with my doctor, and I continued to work even though my stress levels were at their highest point.

Existing for months and even years with stress levels that high can be toxic to your body. I have learned this lesson the hard way, and in fact, I now reject stressful situations for the sake of my health.

In childhood, I was pretty much always a little overweight. But the doctors couldn't understand how because I was so active and strong. And as I grew up, I tried all sorts of diets, only to find out that none ever worked for me. And I had such low energy all the time. At one point, I got into coffee. I got a job working at a coffee shop and thought, "Hey, this is perfect for someone like me. I can drink espresso all day to cope with my lack of energy!" I didn't really know what normal felt like. I thought that being so tired was just a natural state of being. But it wasn't.

Doctors didn't have any answers for me back then; I still don't hear a lot of explanations for thyroid patients from the medical community. One of my clients, functional medicine doctor, Dr. Ben Galyardt, mentioned to me low ferritin (iron) for a prolonged period of time could wreak havoc on the thyroid (I always had low iron!). My experience with doctors would always go this way. I would explain how tired I was all the time and how I found it impossible to lose weight, and they'd just tell me, "You're young, you just need to sleep more," and "You can't really lose weight if you don't eat. Eat more, work out more, eat less, work out more."

I remember going to the gym to do military-caliber workouts for a full month—and not losing even one pound! I'd get really strong, of course, but I'd look and weigh the same while everyone else doing those same workouts was getting thinner.

I knew my body wasn't operating like everyone else's.

I managed to distract myself from the fear and feeling that something was very wrong with me and my lump. While I was busy ignoring it, more blessings came my way in the fall of 2012. I met my soulmate, Dave, and he asked me to marry him a few years later, in the summer of 2016. He was the calm in this life of mine that always felt like a mix of joy and chaos. Meeting Dave was such a blessing. I got pregnant in late 2016 and was fired from my job upon returning from my honeymoon.

I started meditation daily in an attempt to calm my body down. I was aware of the amount of stress my body had been through, and I wanted to make sure I would carry the baby in a place of health. I actually felt an intense amount of relief when I was fired, but I had no idea how much stress I had endured to this point.

When I became pregnant, my lump grew even larger. I went to the endocrinologist, who basically said, "Whoa, how are you growing a baby while this is in your neck? This is not okay."

Dr. Hui at Sunnybrook wanted to do a biopsy and said, "Niki, I think you need to be scared right now; this is serious."

But I didn't believe in being scared. It didn't really sit well with me. I had endured enough and come to the understanding that fear served me in no way.

When I was younger, a nodule in the throat didn't seem like as big of a deal as you'd think. My mother had a nodule in her throat. My cousin in Greece had a nodule in her throat. And then, when I was in my early twenties, they found a nodule in my throat. They basically just monitored it for years. I remember, as a young person, thinking the doctors were crazy for leaving nodules in our throats and that it was such an odd medical system we have here; they just left the nodules there instead of taking them out.

I didn't get the biopsy. I was reluctant to have a procedure like that done while I was carrying a baby. She mentioned to me that the growth seemed far bigger, and she noted that it seemed to be impacted by hormones. She was also afraid that as my pregnancy progressed, it would grow. I am so thankful to Dr. Hui for looking out for my health when she did.

I had often found myself short of breath but had rationalized this by the thought that most pregnant women were out of breath. Going up and down stairs really took the wind out of me. It turned out that I was living on a lot less oxygen than most people due to this growth that was living in my neck.

In lieu of the biopsy, I changed my diet following the advice of my Chinese Medicine Healer. I'm deeply grateful to him for the advice he gave me. Yet, in my heart, I'm sure he knew more was wrong with me than I was ready to face.

* * *

My doctor at the time was very concerned with how relaxed I was about it all. In hindsight, maybe I *was* too relaxed, but it was not cancer for my mother, and in fact, it wasn't cancer for a lot of the women in my family. So, that helped eliminate a lot of my fear.

My obstetrician Dr. Hui asked me, again, to consider a biopsy: "Niki, I'm worried about you. I know you don't want us looking at your thyroid right now, but I need you to know this is serious. Can I have you meet with the surgeon, please? Operations need time to be scheduled, and you don't have time. We know there's a goiter; we just don't know why it's so big and why it's growing."

I agreed and met the surgeon, Dr. Higgins, who strongly advised that I consider the surgery since I had previously declined a biopsy.

I believe that where there is fear, there's an absence of faith. I grew up going to church. We had this amazing Reverend Hedley at Agape Church in Toronto who used to say where there is faith, there's no room for anything else. So, you know, faith first has always guided me.

When I was pregnant, I would run out of breath, literally, just from carrying a child. I would rationalize this by saying, "It's okay. All pregnant women are out of breath! We are carrying something, and this is hard!" I would pause whenever I went down a staircase, say, "Thank you, God," pat my belly, and just keep going. One day I was at TD Bank, and a minister came up to me and asked, "Can I pray over you?" I immediately agreed. I didn't question it. So, all these people were staring at us, and this lady, who's dressed as a Minister, was praying over me and my stomach.

I said, "Thank you, God." when she finished her prayer. That moment was powerful, knowing she was called to pray over me.

Once I gave birth to a healthy baby boy, I was taken by the sudden realization that life was different now.

Now I have to live.

Now I have to be okay.

Now I'm in love with this little munchkin and can't go anywhere.

I have to be okay for him.

So, after I had my son, the surgeon Dr. Higgins at Sunnybrook and I met again. He said, "I'm going to give it to you straight. I'm a busy man. I need to know if you are a 'Yes' or 'No' for surgery. You need it!" And he left the room.

My Chinese doctor had muscle-tested me and said there was cancer in my body.

Here's my advice: When a doctor proposes surgery to remove something, just let them take it out. Do not wait for a biopsy. Just remove it.

So, when Dr. Higgins came back into the room, I said, "Sure."

He said, "Sure is not a definite 'yes.' "

So, I said "Yes" for real and signed the consent forms.

Dr. Higgins said he would see me when he saw me, and just like that, I left the hospital and returned home to my new baby.

Surgeries do take time to set up, so there was a waiting period during which I tried to process it all. Then, I finally got the call. It was a recorded voice that said, "Hello. This is Sunnybrook Hospital. Your surgery is booked."

And then, things got a lot more real. To this day, I am so thankful for these doctors.

The Diagnosis

My son was still young, barely walking, when I arrived at the hospital that crisp fall day. As we drove to the hospital, I remember feeling a lightness of being as I focused my attention only on those things that are beautiful in the world. I found beauty in everything.

I repeated the prayer "Our Father, who art in heaven …" over and over again to help calm my nerves. I also repeated, "I let go and I let God."

It was humbling to realize that I was a new mom and that something serious was going on with my body. I didn't say very much to my husband.

When we reached the hospital, I was given a blue hospital gown and told to change into the hospital gown and wait in the intake area. The room was filled with a bunch of older people. My great-uncle was sitting right beside me in his little hospital gown. And I was like, "Oh, look at that! We're doing this together!"

But that's about all I said because I was in a very deep state of prayer. Moments went by slowly. It dawned on me how important it was to be healthy for my son. Life had taken on a very different meaning for me as a mom. I had so much more to live for and to be healthy for. I was not working at this time but had started my own PR firm. Thankfully, my clients were amazing and very understanding.

The surgery was three hours long.

The surgeon came out and told me, "Niki, it looks good. And I think I even gave you some neck work there."

I said, "Thanks, Higgins!" in the calm, easy way he was accustomed to expecting from me.

When I went back for the results of tests on what had been removed from my throat, I will admit that I was a little bit scared that day. I went into the hospital in a state of prayer, repeating, "Our Father who art in heaven." That's all.

I don't remember walking into the building.

When Dr. Higgins came into the room, he was with another man, a student doctor. My husband presented him with a bottle of wine to say, "Thank you."

He asked me, "Do you want the good news or the bad news?"

For a second or two, I couldn't talk. Then I replied, "Good news or bad news, I can take it. Whatever it is, please just say it."

"Well, the bad news is that it was cancer. And the good news is that I'm good at what I do, and I think I got it all out."

That's when I high-fived him. His reaction was priceless. I don't think it's every day that you tell a person they have cancer and, in return, receive a high five. The student doctor's eyes grew wide with surprise.

I believe that life will always present us with situations, but it's how we respond to them that defines us.

Reality started to hit me. I read the words in the hallway … I was in the cancer unit. Until then, I had not allowed that to scare me or really even enter into my awareness. I felt so much gratitude and said, "Thank you, Lord, for letting me live." I hadn't cherished my body, this temple, in any way. I had let myself get abused.

Months before I went in for surgery, my amazing acupuncturist did a muscle test on me and advised that there was cancer in my body. Mentally, I was prepared for the diagnosis but had not accepted it as my reality or my future. I never said "my cancer." I only said "the cancer." I wasn't owning it.

I was telling God that I learned my lesson. I allowed myself to be treated so terribly for so long, and I did not use my voice. That made me sick. *I* had made myself sick.

I was ready to turn my life around. I felt so much gratitude.

Can we take a minute to acknowledge that my body produced a healthy child while cancer was growing inside of me?!

The body is so miraculous and brilliant and beyond our comprehension.

I asked my friend from church if she had any guidance for me. She connected me to her monk, Father Gheronda. He took a call with me one day while he was sitting on a bench outside a small monastery with my son's name on it.

When I told him my son's name, he reminded me, "God is always talking to us in ways we'll understand. Of course, I'm at St. Nicolas; this is your moment with me." The comfort I got that day is beyond words.

After the call, something in my heart told me everything would somehow be okay.

For me, what worked was to say the "Our Father Thou Art in Heaven" prayer, and just learning to say "Thank you" 100 times a day did the magic. I think the reason I'm still alive is that God is thinking that maybe she could tell other people to say thank you 100 times a day. That's it. As a child, I thought when I grew up I would be a minister of some kind. But just being in a state of gratitude and understanding what we own, what happens to us, is what I was meant to experience.

I spent weeks healing from the surgery in a state of prayer and gratitude. I cut out sugar, I cut out alcohol, and I made very healthy green-based juices to drink. I made soup after soup. I even drank chicken soup broth. I also drank warm ginger honey and lemon tea throughout the day.

I had been told by my Chinese Acupuncturist that my goal was to keep my body warm, and never to drink cold beverages. And the warm liquids were comforting. I took this to heart and drank ginger tea (about three cups) each day. Ginger felt so strong in my hands. Intuitively, I was drawn to continue this process. I still drink ginger tea almost every night!

I still go for annual ultrasounds on my neck. In 2020, I had to go to the appointment with my baby Sofia in tow. I remember having an inward conversation with God that went like this:

"Hey, God? I don't want this reality anymore. No more hospitals, please.

I got the lesson. Can you show me you're with me here? I need to know you heard me."

I went into the exam room and was asked to remove my cross, so I did. Days later, I lost my cross and had almost given up on finding it when my niece Chloe walked up to her mother one day holding it in her hand, "This is Niki's, Mommy."

Her mom consulted a clairvoyant friend of ours, who explained the significance of Chloe finding the necklace: "Niki asked God for a sign, and God directed the sign through Chloe because Chloe would get her aunt's attention." *Doesn't that give you goosebumps?!*

The results of my MRI came by email weeks after the test. I read it on December 24, 2021. It read: "Niki, we love your MRI. Go have a Merry Christmas now!" I felt my shoulders drop, and I let myself feel the relief. I think that was when I cried the most.

As time passes, my life feels like it has more meaning now than ever. I have a daughter, Sofia, who lights up my life, and I have my son, Nicolas, who says the darndest things. My two little chiclets make me want to live an extra one hundred years.

Life After

After the diagnosis, I decided to choose what makes me feel good. If it doesn't feel good, I won't repeat it. I now have immense clarity and can help people. When it doesn't feel good, our gut is like the universe saying, "Hey, don't." And if we could all listen to it, we wouldn't end up in situations where we're sick.

And if it feels good, be grateful for it. If it feels good, it is good *for* you. And, you know, I do think that I have a different perspective after I had cancer. I want to do what makes me feel alive. I want to cherish the seconds, the moments I have with the people I love. I look at everything like it's always for me, in some way. I love grass. I love rain. Rainy days are not sad days; rainy days are beautiful days to be alive. I do understand there's a lot of fear on this Earth, and I don't think fear is helping anybody.

I think if we could have a heavier dose of faith, we could tip the scale of this planet to be very different.

I'm teaching my kids about God the way I know God. My son will tell me he doesn't understand where God is. My response is to just look at the sun and the way it sets and look at the grass and the way it grows; that maybe God is just hidden everywhere, in plain sight. Just trying to explain faith to my kids is helping me so much that when the other day my mom called me with a tech challenge at her restaurant, I suggested that she *pause*. I said, "We're just going to ask God to intervene."

Within no time, she called me back and said, "Oh my goodness, everything just corrected itself!"

Isn't that how everything corrected itself in my life, too? Faith is the only way. There's no other explanation. I feel like I just appealed to God, made a case for life, and acknowledged all that I'd done wrong. I said a million thank-yous for learning the lesson and taking responsibility for how I had allowed cancer to be in my body, enduring so much stress.

In the hospital, I often asked the nurses if they were okay. The nurses all seemed tired and weary. One nurse shared that they'd had a young man in hospital recently and they were still mourning him. He did not tell his mommy he had cancer. He told his mom it was pneumonia. He'd just had his mom with him for weeks, taking care of him, and she wondered why he wasn't getting better, and he didn't want her to be sad. *Oh my God, what a story!* These poor nurses told me story after story like this.

I just want to tell the world that these nurses, even though they are there to take care of *us*, they all need a hug. They need "thank-yous." Thank them for what they do because, emotionally, the work is exhausting beyond words. How do they release stories like these? People thought it was crazy I was letting nurses open up to me.

What better gift can we give our kids than the *inner knowing* that if you turn to the right thing, you'll be okay? That if you pray you feel calmer. And it's true, even in this world, that can scare the **** out of us! Really! That's the only way. My beautiful friend called me one day and asked if we could discuss my experience. She asked me why her friend with the same health scare was having a really hard time with it all. I remember closing my eyes and wondering how to send this human strength. I explained that the only thing that really changed my life was asking God to take the lead.

The vitamins, the food, all of that was positive, but asking God for help was how I generally stayed calm. In the end, I sent her friend some of the superfoods I was taking but truly just prayed to God she would be okay and would be humble enough to try faith on for a minute. I knew it would calm her.

I have also cut out toxic people from my life and set up boundaries for what I would accept moving forward. I work with clients who are on the same energy level as me. I realized my life really was given a second chance because of cancer and because of God. And the feeling of gratitude I feel because of it grows stronger and stronger every day.

I planted my first vegetable garden in 2018, and my father asked if I was crazy (because I had a lot going on). My joy came from eating what I harvested, and that has become a tradition for me. It reminds me constantly of the earth's abundance that exists despite us humans.

I did a cancer walk one weekend in 2022, and they started the event by talking about how many people had died. I made a mental note to bring headphones the following year and start the walk after this part. I didn't want to focus on how many died, but celebrate the people who have survived and come for the walk! Let's celebrate being alive, and let's celebrate the success of coming out of the other side with a different perspective. I believe that is a miracle, a gift.

People sometimes don't understand me because it sounds a little bit like believing in unicorns. When you've crossed over that hump, you know that you have two choices. I can go back to being numb, stressed, and unaware, or I can be calm and grateful. And manage it delicately. Manage the body delicately.

I recommend having mercy on your soul. I think that when you've seen somebody pass away, you understand that it's just the breath. So we are about a breath between life and death. We tend to be hard on our bodies. We treat this body like it can take so much. At some point, it breaks if you are not aligned with your emotional, mental, and physical place and really working to stay calm.

I was never somebody to pop an Advil or Tylenol. When I was younger, to help me manage my weight, my doctor recommended birth control pills. I took it for a week, and my body said no and refused to take it. Even then, I had an awareness that I could not do this to my body.

After cancer, I think my prescription is to say "thank you" twenty-five times a day. *Thank you, thank you, thank you.* That's all. Just *thank you.* And I'm told by people that I'm very connected now, connected to my own inner intelligence. I listen to my gut. It's not perfected yet, but I'm honing the ability to *just listen and say thank you.* And as a result, I feel like the universe always has my back—and your back and everyone's back. *If* we're humble enough to listen. When we're quiet, we can hear that voice.

The funny thing is, at my PR business, I represent two doctors and one Naturopath. I don't think this is accidental. I think I understand their true intentions, and I know the job of a doctor is exhausting. I follow some very interesting people and live a pretty unique life. My thoughts around health are still that we are 100% responsible for how we handle and heal from what happens to us, and that stress is not a natural state of being. I accomplish so much more from a place of joy than I ever did from a place of high stress.

People comment on my demeanor. They say I'm very calm. I don't take anything personally. If it feels wrong, I allow myself to freely decline. I also cherish days. I love mornings. I love rainfall. I love life. I am so thankful that I'm alive. I'm also the person in the room who does not panic when others freak out. I figure out the solution, and I ask God to intervene if I cannot figure it out.

I pray twenty times a day. Before I have a meeting, after I have a meeting, before I drive, and before my kids leave for school …

My little guy asked how I heard God. I explained that I meditate, I go inward and I listen. When I'm quiet, divine guidance comes to me clearly.

After my surgery, I couldn't talk for a few weeks. I had the feeling of having lost my voice. Fisherman's Friend lozenges saved me. I always had one in my mouth. I felt like they were opening up my air passageways. *The Medical Medium* became something I was avidly reading. I read all of *The Medical Medium* books, and I started welcoming celery juice and fruit back into my life. You would see me making crazy healing soups. Lots of chicken broth, beef broth, and sweet potatoes. I think now my kids eat really interesting food because *I believe like my Greek predecessors that food is health.*

In 2021, I bought like 100 bottles of vitamin C and gave them out during the holidays. What better gift could I give than the gift of good health? What could be better than vitamin C during the pandemic? And if you take it, your immune system will be strong, or you'll know someone like me loves you.

I just want everyone to understand what I've learned: that bliss is the natural state of being. Bliss and gratitude are what we should all aspire to. We don't have room for anything else.

For people experiencing cancer right now, I just want to say that *food is medicine*, and stress has to go. And I really lean toward receiving healing through different parts of the world. I allowed Western medicine to operate on me, and I took thyroid medicine, but then I *also* took my Chinese doctor's advice. I do believe that everything we put in our body is either medicine or it's hurtful. For example, stress is hurtful, and so is sugar. Sugar doesn't love us—it is sweet for a second in our mouths, but I believe that it debilitates the body. And the body, I believe, knows how to tell us when something's wrong.

Some people might ask, why did you need surgery if you have so much faith in God? I think God is the one who told me to get surgery.

It was in the middle of the night. A nurse came to me to help with my bandages, and I was nursing at the time.

He said, "Oh, Mama, you're doing this too. Okay, I see you. I'm sorry, I'm going to have to clean you up. You need a different hospital gown."

I looked down and felt so embarrassed. I didn't have a voice, and I was leaking milk. I thought to myself, *You are not cool anymore.* I remember my husband apologizing to the nurse. And the nurse said, "Don't you be sorry for your wife being so giving of herself, my friend; she is still bleeding." It was a really interesting moment to cherish my body. To grow a baby with cancer is miraculous, but until that moment, I didn't realize how much I had been giving.

When Nicolas was born, he was my healthy little Frank Sinatra—he came out like a little old man. My son is a little angel. He feels like he is my protector. He is very protective of his mummy. I cheer him on because I'm his biggest fan. I think if it were not for being pregnant with him, I would never have received any kind of guidance or treatment for my neck, because when I heard the first time that doctors were not concerned about it, I thought this was something I had to live with. As a result, I didn't advocate for myself. I needed to learn that. My son came to save me totally. He's so cute, and he's wise. Anything I adjust, he adjusts. If it's green juice, he drinks it. If it's ginger tea, he drinks it. He's not sure about it; he doesn't like the flavor, but if I drink it, he drinks it. I have a great bond with him.

When Nicolas came out, I said, "You're too special. You need a buddy!"

My husband didn't think that my body could endure another pregnancy. He didn't think it was healthy to have another baby. And I was determined that Nicolas would not be alone. So, we had another child, our cute little Sofia. And Sofia protects Nicolas. It's like this cute little bond. She's like his little mommy. And for these two little people, I think if I could just teach them about God the way I know God, they are going to show the world something different.

My daughter and my son don't know what life was like for me, before them. To me, they are the reason I made it this far. I have so many lessons to learn. So many things to share with them. I want to be their guiding light toward faith, a faith that's kept me here and given me so much perspective on life. I'm so thankful for living this life intentionally. The same God that listens to me daily is listening to *you* ... if you are open.

I'm here to tell you that you will keep going. In whatever form, you *will* keep going. You are not forgettable. I will never forget what facing death felt like, and therefore, I know that living life is like getting to enjoy a sweetness that I know doesn't last forever—nothing does. So, I'm just making the most out of it *now*.

During moments when fear crept in, I read this prayer over and over again and felt the calm take over, and I want to leave it with you:

Our Father, who art in heaven,
hallowed be Thy name;
thy kingdom come; Thy will be done;
on earth as it is in heaven.
Give us this day our daily bread.
And forgive us our trespasses, as we forgive those who trespass against us.
And lead us not into temptation; but deliver us from evil.
For Thine is the kingdom, the power and the glory,
for ever and ever.
Amen

NIKI PAPAIOANNOU

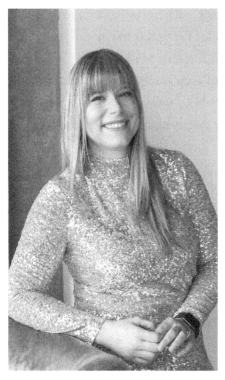

Niki Papaioannou is the founder of Niki Inc., a Toronto-based publicity firm. A mother of two, a survivor, and a philanthropist, Niki is always incorporating a nonprofit approach to 20% of Niki Inc.'s lead PR initiatives. It is through these initiatives that she works with superstars and entrepreneurs who want to improve the state of the planet and tell their unique stories. Niki Inc. supports the BIPOC community through her employment selections and her work with Foodpreneur Lab.

Niki Papaioannou spent over ten years in senior marketing roles with a focus on the casual dining/restaurant sector, where she honed her passion for food and storytelling into successful publicity strategies and marketing campaigns. Her collaborative approach to knowing the audience and speaking to them in their own vernacular garnered Niki great acclaim within the industry.

Niki took extensive media-relations training while working at these North American restaurant chains and decided after ten amazing years that it was time to branch out on her own.

Niki is a contributing author of *Business Hacks: Growth Secrets They Don't Want You to Know BOOK 2*, released in 2021.

Niki is the co-producer of a radio show called *Solving Healthcare with*

Dr. K (https://sauga960am.ca/on-air-hosts/). She proudly represents Dr. Kwadwo Kyeremanteng and functional doctor Ben Galyardt and works with the Greek hotel, The Cretan Dream.

One non-profit that Niki Inc. proudly represents is called Foodpreneur Lab. They are the only Canadian Black woman-founded and led non-profit with a fierce national mandate to advance racial and gender equity by supporting Canadian Startup and Scale Up food businesses. To learn more about Niki, go to *www.torontopragency.com.*

NIKI PAPAIOANNOU

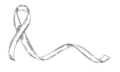

CHAPTER NINE

AWAKENING THE MIND'S POTENTIAL

by Tania Kolar

*Miracles are natural and when they do not occur
something has gone wrong.*
—*Helen Schucman, A Course in Miracles*

A soul retrieval journey, meant to reconnect the lost parts of my soul, might have saved my life. My friend Stephanie, while completing her Master Shamanic Practitioner certification, offered me a soul retrieval session to finalize her training. While I had previously experimented with alternative healing techniques like reiki, EFT tapping, timeline therapy, and past life regression, a soul retrieval was uncharted territory for me. Shamanic principles suggest that soul loss from trauma can often lead to illness, manifesting as chronic depression, post-traumatic stress syndrome, immune deficiency issues, or persistent grief. Given my past experiences with grief, trauma, and PTSD, it seemed likely that my soul might be fragmented. I wasn't certain, but if any part of me was astray, I yearned to reclaim it. With an open mind, I delved deeper and agreed to a session.

Weeks later, as I lay on a massage table, I embarked on an enlightening journey. Though the session lasted an hour, it felt fleeting. Stephanie recounted her visions and her discoveries about my soul, leaving me feeling serene and rejuvenated. She mentioned witnessing a past life of mine that influenced my present—one where I was an overlooked young girl, taught to conceal her gifts. Most startlingly, she intimated that I had a lump in my breast and urged me to consult a doctor. I pondered on how she could have possibly known.

The term "shaman" translates to "one who sees in the dark." I often wish I had this uncanny ability to perceive amidst obscurity. For almost two years, I had harbored a secret lump in my breast. Without revealing this, I probed Stephanie further, inquiring which breast housed the lump. She instantly pointed to the left. The accuracy of her response was jolting. It seemed the soul retrieval not only reconnected me to parts of my soul but also illuminated a pressing physical concern. Perhaps Stephanie truly did possess the ability to see in the dark.

Universe: message received.

Prior to the soul retrieval, warning signs had appeared: a changing shape, bruising, and unusual discharge from my breast. Despite the indicators, I had been in denial. The persistent aches, the fatigue—they were all screams for attention. But the shadow of COVID and the fear of bad news kept me from consulting a doctor. My niece, Sarah, had also faced a significant health scare due to a breast lump. Though benign, it served as a stark reminder for me, one which I chose to ignore until the session with Stephanie. The very next day, I set an appointment with my family doctor. After an ultrasound, I was promptly sent for a mammogram. The ensuing results were bleak. The mass was identified, and my doctor later informed me of its abnormal cells and notable size—roughly five centimeters in diameter. While I hoped for the best, a visit to the Women's Cancer Centre at Credit Valley Hospital culminated in a life-altering revelation: I had cancer.

Though intuition had hinted at the truth, the reality, when vocalized, was still numbing. The information overload was overwhelming, yet there was a peculiar relief in finally naming my ailment. After the diagnosis, I awaited further tests, recalling the strength and resilience my father exhibited during his battle with stage IV stomach cancer.

Would I share this news with my family or friends? And if so, who should hear it first?

The weight of these questions made everything feel even more surreal. Driving away from the hospital, I sought solace in the Ho'oponopono Prayer, a Hawaiian mantra of love, apology, forgiveness, and gratitude.

I'm sorry. Please forgive me. Thank you. I love you.

Its comforting repetitions brought me momentary peace.

This tranquility resonated with the remarkable journey undertaken by clinical psychologist Dr. Hew Len as he collaborated with patients at the Hawaii State Hospital, individuals classified as criminally insane. Dr. Len's approach defied convention, rooted in a meticulous examination of their medical histories, enriched by a profound and transformative practice. Instead of adhering to traditional therapeutic methods, Dr. Hew Len quietly repeated the powerful mantra: "I love you. I'm sorry. Please forgive me. Thank you." This unique methodology would eventually yield extraordinary results.

Dr. Hew Len's approach transcended the ordinary boundaries of healing. He held a profound belief that his work was not a direct healing of his patients but rather a process of cleansing the part of himself that recognized them. Articulating this perspective, he conveyed, "I was merely purifying the part of me that I shared with them. Everything that appears in our life is our responsibility." This philosophy underscored the interconnectedness of all human experiences and highlighted the transformative power of self-awareness and personal responsibility within the healing process.

In essence, Dr. Hew Len's practice was not solely aimed at alleviating the suffering of his patients but also represented a profound journey of self-discovery and personal growth. It underscored the idea that healing extends beyond the individual to encompass the broader web of human existence.

Throughout my car ride, I recited this prayer continuously, echoing Dr. Hew Len's approach by accepting responsibility for my cancer diagnosis. Just as he sought to heal the part of himself shared with his patients, I aimed to heal and accept my own journey.

I'd previously viewed myself as immune to the disease, but reality proved otherwise. I believed this challenge was part of the Universe's grand design, so I embraced it. I've realized that challenges often bring unexpected gifts. Thus, I committed to seeking the gift this experience might offer without waiting for years or decades as I did in past situations.

I saw my cancer diagnosis as a nudge, directing me to address unsettled aspects within myself. It felt like a tangible reminder of unresolved emotional wounds. My body carried the weight of past traumas—decades of pent-up hurt, anger, fear, and sadness, which had now manifested as a disease.

Several years prior, I had been brutally attacked in an underground parking lot. The sheer violence of the incident led the police to initially suspect that it was a targeted attack. I had kept the ordeal private, not allowing others in, standing alone even in the hospital's emergency room. That traumatic experience had opened my eyes to my self-limiting beliefs and patterns. Over the years, I began sharing my story, culminating in writing a book to aid others through their own adversities. To me, this cancer felt like another chance—a call to prioritize my well-being and let others be there for me.

The night after the diagnosis, a dream filled my sleep—faces laden with diverse emotions, from fear to rage, seemingly symbolizing long-suppressed feelings now rising to the surface.

After weeks of introspection, I shared the news of my diagnosis with my family. It was a challenging conversation, particularly with my younger relatives, and it brought me to tears. One sibling labeled the revelation as "brutal."

In response, I offered a different perspective: "Let's not classify it as brutal. This journey will be what I choose to make of it." If I refused to view my situation as "brutal," why should anyone else view it so?

Human nature often inclines toward negativity. However, what if we deliberately trained ourselves to recognize the positives? Many past worries, when revisited, appear to have been exaggerated by overthinking.

Embracing the present moment and immersing ourselves in inner stillness can liberate us from the shackles of negative thoughts.

Reflecting upon my cancer journey, I'm overwhelmed by the support I received—from close ones to strangers. My niece Ally, an angel by my side, took on the role of driving me to all my chemotherapy appointments, offering not only her time but her unwavering love and care. This warmth taught me that seeking help isn't a sign of weakness. Initially, accepting help felt awkward, but I soon grasped the power of community support. Cancer can feel isolating, but the collective goodwill of others can be a potent salve.

In the past, I would hesitate to express my requirements, and I was reluctant to disclose my strict organic nutrition plan during treatment. But, through my journey, I learned the importance of specificity—it not only enables others to assist more effectively but also ensures my needs are met.

To all who are reading this, if you find yourself navigating through challenging times, please remember that it's perfectly okay to reach out and ask for help. You are not alone, and there is support available to you. Always hold onto the belief that you are whole, deserving, loved, remarkable, and complete.

During those moments when your spirits may falter, consider prompting yourself with empowering questions.

For instance:

- "What can I glean from this experience that can contribute to my personal growth?"
- "What is the hidden gift in this situation that I may not have noticed yet?"
- "How does facing this challenge empower me to extend a helping hand to others going through their own crisis?"
- "What actions can I take to cultivate happiness and contentment in this very moment?"

When I met my oncologist, she expressed confidence that the cancer had spread, suggesting an underarm biopsy to confirm. The news left me deflated. The doctor performing the biopsy inquired about my oncologist's reasons for recommending one and if I had any other abnormal test results. I mentioned a physical exam had detected swollen lymph nodes. Wishing to consult my oncologist to ensure a consistent approach, he called her. Following their discussion, he informed me there was no need for the biopsy as everything appeared normal.

It felt like a miracle.

* * *

My treatment journey began with several rounds of chemotherapy, which were followed by surgery. After undergoing additional tests, including a bone density test and MRI to ensure my suitability for chemotherapy, I embarked on a comprehensive treatment plan that combined both traditional and alternative therapies. I always encourage others to conduct their research and trust their instincts when navigating medical decisions.

On the morning of my first chemotherapy session, a profound sense of calm embraced me. I vividly remembered the song "Angel of the Morning" playing in my mind and the invigorating walk I had taken the previous night.

After completing the initial round of chemotherapy, I noticed that my tumor appeared smaller. I found myself contemplating whether my alternative healing practices were genuinely effective or if it was just wishful thinking. However, my doubts were dispelled during a follow-up appointment with both the oncologist and surgeon, who confirmed the tumor's reduction. This news left me absolutely elated.

The tumor symbolized years of neglect, accumulating layer upon layer, demanding my attention much like a persistent child.

The expression "Live like you are dying" encourages us to embrace life to the fullest. While I value the sentiment behind it, I tend to favor the notion of "Living as if you are fully alive," cherishing each moment without dwelling on the past or worrying about the future.

Regrettably, a chemotherapy session was slated for Christmas Eve. I had eagerly anticipated the family gathering, especially after the previous year's COVID-19 lockdown. Then, it occurred to me that I could request a rescheduling. The shift was simpler than anticipated, emphasizing the power within seeking what one needs.

Cancer has been a profound teacher in my life, imparting invaluable lessons about the importance of self-care and emotional processing. Through this challenging journey, I've come to realize that happiness doesn't solely rely on perfect circumstances. Life's inherent messiness should not be a barrier to our happiness. In response, I made a steadfast commitment to approach my cancer diagnosis with a positive outlook, embracing whatever challenges it presented.

I've come to regard my experience with cancer as a blessing in disguise. It has compelled me to engage in deep introspection and has provided me with a platform to extend my support to others facing similar circumstances.

When we manage to break free from limited thinking and rise above negativity, we unlock our inherent strengths and discover the wellspring of resources within us. This journey reminds us that even in the face of adversity, there is a reservoir of resilience and untapped potential waiting to be harnessed.

I had long used food as an emotional crutch, trying to reconnect with my late parents and relive familiar comforts. Upon closer scrutiny, I discerned a pattern: stress and anxiety triggered junk food cravings. This revelation prompted a change in my habits.

My previous habits reflected self-sabotage. Despite awareness of the harm certain foods posed, I indulged. *Why this self-defeating pattern?* Stress consistently led to poor decisions. With a deep-rooted desire for comfort and love, I needed to confront and process these emotions rather than seek fleeting solace in food.

The words of Dr. Mincolla, a nutritional therapist and quantum energy healer, resonated deeply with me. Recognizing his wisdom, I committed to his nutrition plan. Life's fragility and our innate power became evident to me, prompting an unwavering resolve to maintain this nutritional discipline. Dr. Mincolla urged me to trust my intuition. Having previously overlooked my body's signals, I now heeded his counsel, aligning with my newfound awareness.

* * *

Dear reader, what immediate steps can you undertake to elevate your mental and physical well-being amid health challenges? If your body seems uncooperative, how might you mentally lift your spirits? Obsessing over future outcomes can induce anxiety; thus, anchoring your attention to the present moment is pivotal.

* * *

Cancer, albeit daunting, can illuminate one's life. The diagnosis can spur a compelling urge toward a healthier lifestyle, refining your values and focal points. Achieving profound clarity and a tranquil mind can dispel uncertainties. Meditation can be a powerful tool, allowing you to let go of the need to control external circumstances and find inner peace by fully immersing yourself in the present moment.

By immersing yourself fully in the present moment, you lay the foundation for the inner peace that is rightfully yours to claim. With a surge of determination coursing through me, I made a resolute decision to prioritize my health and well-being. Each day I applied makeup and, at times, I even used self-tanner to counteract the pallor of my skin. Maintaining my pre-cancer style, I'd don heels, dresses, and earrings for my chemotherapy sessions. This routine not only uplifted my spirits but also provided a semblance of normalcy in a challenging time. Having friends who were simultaneously navigating the labyrinth of cancer was a tremendous source of comfort. Our shared experiences, along with the mutual encouragement and understanding we offered one another, formed a tightly-knit support network that guided us through this challenging journey together.

Despite the frequent bouts of nausea, fatigue, and other debilitating symptoms, my determination to seize every moment's potential joy remained unshaken. Many remarked on my surprisingly upbeat demeanor and appearance, even amidst numerous chemo cycles. This kind of feedback, along with my oncologist's genuine astonishment upon nearly failing to recognize me as a patient in a hallway, served as a powerful boost to my spirits.

To incorporate some activity, I opted for stairs whenever feasible. Although the hospital's layout required frequent movement between levels, I persevered at my own pace, occasionally resorting to elevators when necessary. Recognizing and respecting one's boundaries is paramount.

Your body possesses inherent recuperative abilities. By invoking the body's wisdom, one can dispel ailments and discard what no longer benefits you. Embracing positive thoughts can unleash creativity, curiosity, and courage, propelling your self-belief. As an exceptional being in a wondrous world, you're endowed with spiritual riches. Everything essential lies within you.

Set healing intentions but remain unattached to specific outcomes. Allow yourself the grace to unwind.

* * *

While my initial intention was to exercise daily, the overwhelming fatigue that accompanied my journey with cancer soon became an undeniable presence. My ambition clashed with the very real constraints of my body. Over time, I began to release the self-imposed pressure of constant activity and instead embraced the paramount importance of health and recuperation. I learned the vital lesson of recognizing and respecting my current physical state, understanding that self-care and healing were equally essential components of my journey.

* * *

Contemplate: What insights might arise if you viewed your predicament through the lens of wisdom rather than trepidation? What valuable lessons are concealed within your experiences, waiting to be uncovered?

The Challenge of Side Effects

Cancer treatment side effects are prevalent, and I experienced a myriad of them, including the loss of my hair, eyebrows, eyelashes, and toenails. Unable to alter these side effects, I sought lessons within them.

After my second chemotherapy cycle, my hair largely fell out within days. This was when the reality of cancer truly sank in. I trimmed the sparse remaining patches as short as I could. Soon after, I chose to shave off the remnants. The initial phase, with hair falling out in clumps and a bathroom bin filled with my hair, was the most distressing. But once I was entirely bald, there was a strange sense of liberation. I was unsettled by the patchy hair, which served as a constant reminder of my declining health. A smooth bald appearance was preferable over confronting a sickly reflection in the mirror.

I resolved to get a wig. However, finding one that resonated with me proved challenging. Despite visiting several specialized wig stores, some boasting over 500 varieties, I found no match. After trying numerous options at one store, the assistant remarked, "We've exhausted all our options." This was disheartening. Thankfully, based on a friend's suggestion, a salon crafted a custom wig mirroring my natural hair.

Losing my hair was far from a delightful experience. However, rather than dwelling on my feelings about the situation, I began to question whether I could cope with it. Coping with hair loss is undeniably challenging, but such introspection can reveal unexpected reserves of resilience. It's essential to recall that despite the outward changes, your inner essence remains unchanged. Recognizing this can be crucial in accepting your altered appearance and acknowledging your enduring strength. During an outing with my dear friend Greta, as I wore my wig for the first time, a young man complimented my "hair." Initially, I thought he was jesting or realized it was a wig. However, his sincerity was evident, and I expressed gratitude. His genuine praise alleviated my wig-related anxieties.

Neuropathy caused pain in my feet and toes, which, thanks to the chemo cycles, were dry and ridged. I kept my nails trimmed, as the chemotherapy rendered them dry, indented, and susceptible to snags, splits, and breaks.

My big toenails took months to fully detach, turning discolored and deformed in the interim. The prospect of losing my toenails was unnerving, but once they fell off, new ones began to grow. Astonishingly, the emerging nails were robust and healthy. This transformation highlighted that occasionally, outcomes we dread can be superior to our initial circumstances. My reluctance to accept the loss of my nails transformed into gratitude for the renewed growth.

Change, particularly when it manifests as unforeseen losses or challenges, can be daunting. Yet, if we approach it with an adaptable mindset, we might discover that the ensuing outcomes surpass our previous circumstances.

The Upside of Side Effects

Change, even as a result of side effects, can be positive. I've compiled a short list below of what I've discovered about the upside of side effects.

- **Hair loss:** The knowledge that despite what physical changes you experience, your soul remains unchanged, and you are still whole and complete.
- **Nail problems:** Symbolic rebirth. A renewal. A shedding of the old. Sometimes, life has a better plan than what we planned for ourselves. We can't move to a higher ground when we are hanging on to a lower level.

- **Bruising:** An outward manifestation of the emotional wounds that linger beneath the surface. A reminder that physical and emotional healing takes time. Have patience with yourself and the process you are going through.
- **Changes in appetite:** Opportunity to reassess the foods you've been eating and take better care of yourself by eating healthier.
- **Body changes:** Recognition of the magnificence of your body.
- **Fatigue:** A necessary reboot, reset, and pause from the chaos of life. The opportunity to make yourself a priority, to get plenty of rest, and to give yourself permission to heal.

For years, I practiced gratitude. But my bout with cancer intensified this sense of thankfulness. I'm thankful for the unexpected benefits of side effects and for avoiding other potential complications.

Before my diagnosis, I yearned for thicker hair. As I began losing it, I wished it back just as it had been. Now, I'm profoundly grateful it's regrowing.

I've rekindled my appreciation for life's minutiae. Once, having my nails done was a professional necessity, and while initially enjoyable, it later felt like an obligation. Post-chemotherapy, my first manicure became an event I eagerly anticipated. It underscored the joy in everyday moments and the danger of taking them for granted.

Advocating for oneself in the realm of healthcare is of paramount importance. I implore everyone to be proactive by asking questions, conducting research, and trusting their instincts. When I received a stage II diagnosis and was advised to undergo a double mastectomy, radiation, and several years of hormone therapy, I couldn't shake the feeling that some of these treatments were excessive for my situation. Despite understanding the medical rationale, I remained unconvinced and exercised my agency to opt out of some of these treatments. It's all too common for people to silence themselves out of fear of judgment when their instincts diverge from medical recommendations.

On the day of my surgery, a porter mistakenly left me outside the wrong operating room. In that unexpected moment, not realizing I was in the wrong place, I found solace playing Wordle on my phone to pass the time. Despite the mix-up, the porter's genuine kindness shone through. When I finally entered the correct surgical area, I couldn't help but notice the date: 2/2/22, a palindromic sequence that I viewed as an angelic sign, providing comfort. Interestingly, upon awakening post-surgery, my mind amusingly engaged in a virtual game of Wordle, illustrating the power of the subconscious and the significance of mindful thought.

Like many, I was perpetually caught up in the busyness of life. That all changed when the combination of fatigue, cognitive issues, and sleep deprivation forced me to slow down. Recognizing my need for healing, I made a conscious decision to pause.

It was during this time that someone asked me about my hobbies, and I realized that my connection to joy outside of work had waned. Cancer forced me to reprioritize, emphasizing the importance of finding enjoyment beyond my career. Since then, I've made a solemn vow to savor life's moments, recommitting to my loved ones and reopening my long-closed heart chakra.

After my second surgery, I experienced a rejuvenation I hadn't anticipated. While the physical changes were evident, the internal metamorphosis was profound. With each medical intervention, I envisioned reshaping myself, experiencing a spiritual renaissance, and cultivating a deep-seated drive to become the very best version of myself.

From my father, who faced terminal illness with joy, I learned the art of finding happiness under any circumstance. When I was diagnosed, his strength buoyed me during my treatments. Reflecting on his ordeal evoked sorrow, but it also granted empathy. Experiencing something similar fosters deeper understanding.

Cancer, in many ways, heightened my self-awareness. It disrupted the cells of my body, much like how my self-isolation was disrupting the natural rhythm of life. This journey underscored the intrinsic human need for connection. By holding back my trust from others, I was effectively denying myself love.

This profound experience cultivated a profound sense of empathy and compassion within me, even for those who had previously betrayed my trust. It became evident that deep truths reside within us, often defying the limitations of language. Through my connection with this inner wisdom, I nurtured a deeper understanding of both myself and the world around me.

A pivotal lesson I embraced was the importance of not taking things personally. It's tempting to interpret others' actions as directed at us or as signs of their indifference. However, it's essential to realize that often, their actions aren't about us. They might be grappling with their own challenges, stress, or may simply be unaware of how we feel. It's crucial not to jump to conclusions. If others fall short of our expectations, it's our task to look after our own well-being. At the heart of it all, our relationship with ourselves is the most significant.

Confronting mortality accentuates the value of time and the choices we make regarding its use. How do we wish to spend each moment of our finite lives? What legacy do we aim to bequeath to our descendants?

Now, having lived through decades of ups and downs, I feel my journey has only just begun. There's so much more I aspire to achieve. I believe that every experience, whether perceived as good or bad, unfolds for a reason, directed by some higher orchestration. My mission is clear: to uplift humanity and augment collective consciousness by sharing my journey, talents, insights, and lessons learned.

I firmly believe that life's most challenging moments hold the potential to transform into profound blessings, leading us toward the core of our authentic selves. Among the 7.8 billion individuals on this planet, each person occupies a unique and invaluable space in the intricate tapestry of existence. My life's purpose revolves around guiding individuals to rediscover their innate magnificence, empowering them to embrace their distinctive gifts and radiate their brilliance.

As I reflect on my journey, I'm reminded of my first encounter with

Dr. Mincolla, who was a guest on my radio show. You may recall him from earlier in this chapter, where I shared how I followed his nutritional advice. Our initial meeting took place when he was promoting his acclaimed book and documentary, *The Way of Miracles*, which showcased his patients' incredible healing journeys. Little did I know that during the filming of those miracles, he would become a living testament to his own healing methods, recovering from a paralyzing disease.

Our initial connection almost slipped through the cracks. You see, our conversation had originally been scheduled for a few weeks prior, but due to unforeseen travel, I had to reschedule. As it turns out, this rescheduling played a pivotal role in our story. It was during one of those precious moments between segments that I confided in him, expressing my hope for a personal miracle.

What unfolded from that point was nothing short of miraculous. Dr. Mincolla, now not just a respected figure but a trusted confidant, began guiding me with tailored nutritional advice. He also emphasized the importance of intuition, a lesson he had personally learned through his own journey. Having previously overlooked my own intuition, I now found myself finely attuned to it, understanding the profound significance of listening to one's inner voice.

Life's fragility and our innate power became evident to me, prompting an unwavering resolve to maintain this nutritional discipline. Dr. Mincolla urged me to trust my intuition, and having once overlooked my body's signals, I now heeded his counsel, aligning with my newfound awareness.

I acknowledge that perspectives on alternative therapies may vary. Therefore, my heartfelt advice is simple: trust your instincts, follow your gut. Your intuition, a wellspring of hidden wisdom, has the capacity to unveil concealed pathways and illuminate your journey forward.

I hold that miracles surround us, yet our ego often obstructs our perception of them. Quieting this egoistic chatter grants us access to a realm where true miracles manifest—a space filled with self-healing and endless possibilities.

As a peak-performance mindset coach and empowerment advocate, I help individuals rewire their thought patterns, direct their focus, and unlock their utmost potential. I've felt the weight of unworthiness, negativity, and life's trials. However, I also understand the transformative power of intentional thought.

The conscious mind, our thinking center, possesses the ability to reason, analyze, decide, and discern. This part of our mind remains acutely aware of our surroundings and can recall memories or envision possible futures. Consequently, by deliberately directing our conscious thoughts, we can mold our desired outcomes. If left unguided, however, the subconscious mind can take the reins, much like a car set to autopilot.

The subconscious mind faithfully follows the conscious mind's lead. Unlike the conscious mind, which analyzes, rationalizes, and chooses, the subconscious accepts and stores information without judgment. It believes whatever it's told, regardless of the information's veracity. By using positive affirmations, you can reprogram the subconscious mind to alter your vibrations and shift your state. Affirmations are potent tools to counteract prevailing negative thought patterns.

The subconscious exists in the present. It doesn't dwell on the past or future. Anything you convey to your conscious mind will imprint upon your subconscious. Serving as the repository of your beliefs, the subconscious records every thought and action. It's essential to remain alert to negative patterns, as thoughts engender emotions. Prolonged negative emotional states can potentially culminate in disease. However, by harnessing the power of the subconscious, you can make it an ally in your healing process.

The Reticular Activating System (RAS) acts as the brain's filter, sifting out irrelevant information to allow only the crucial bits through. As the principle goes, energy goes where focus flows. By emphasizing positive experiences, you condition your brain to recognize more of such instances. Your mind doesn't differentiate between reality and imagination. The objective is to vividly visualize your desires, enabling your mind to transform these aspirations into reality. On days I felt unwell, I would conjure images of my healthier self, tapping into the sensations of well-being.

My path to improved health commenced with an exploratory soul retrieval, guiding me to reclaim fragmented parts of my soul. This experience illuminated the trapped emotions within, which I discerned were culprits for my ailments. Stephanie, a dear friend and visionary guide, played a pivotal role by urging me to promptly get a lump in my breast examined. Without her timely counsel, I might have procrastinated, and the cancer could have progressed, for it doesn't wait.

May you, like the Shaman who perceives through the darkness, tread forward with enlightened clarity, fortifying both mind and body, and may you embrace your own miraculous journey.

TANIA KOLAR

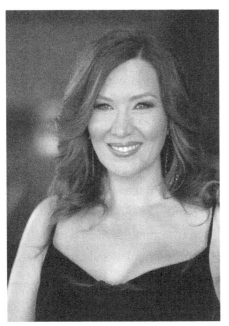

Tania Kolar is a force to be reckoned with in the realm of personal development and peak performance. As a highly sought-after peak performance mindset coach, she has empowered countless individuals and organizations to reach new heights. Tania boasts an impressive portfolio, serving as an international speaker, bestselling author, distinguished radio and TV personality, and the president and founder of Ignite Life Mastery Inc.

In addition, Tania captivates audiences as the host of *The Mindset Mentor* radio show, where her influential voice on mindset and transformation has earned her well-deserved recognition. Her bestselling book, *Breaking The Stupid Mold*, provides readers with actionable, step-by-step strategies to identify and overcome negative patterns and limiting beliefs, enabling them to wholeheartedly embrace life.

At the heart of her mission lies an unwavering commitment to elevating human potential on a global scale. Through her company, Ignite Life Mastery Inc., Tania is dedicated to inspiring entrepreneurs and organizations to reach their next level of human performance. She is a two-time Halo award winner, receiving the highly-coveted Amber Price Spiritual Award of Excellence, a testament to her exceptional impact and contributions to the spiritual community.

Tania is also a prominent figure in the luxury real estate market, using her unique approach to help clients align their mindset with their dream homes. Her dedication to making a profound difference resonates through her personalized coaching, inspiring seminars, captivating live events, and the educational platform of her online academy. Tania Kolar's unwavering commitment to impacting the masses and unlocking boundless potential solidify her position as a true catalyst for transformation. To learn more about Tania, please visit *www.taniakolar.com.*

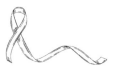

CHAPTER TEN

CANCER RIDE

by Catherine Clark

The Dark Gift: Perhaps our true mission in this life is to harness the power, light, and inner resources in adversity so that we may emerge from darkness with newfound insight, strength, and prosperity. For if we can see our inner and outer experiences with a fresh new perspective, even something as horrible as cancer might be viewed as a Gift in a Dark Package.
—*Catherine Clark, Gifts in Dark Packages*

When we are no longer able to change a situation,
we are challenged to change ourselves.
—*Viktor Frankl*

I could not breathe. I was terrified that if I lost my composure even for one second, it would be my last. I had asked my dad to pull over at least five times.

The color had started to drain from his face as he asked, "What's the exit to the airport?" He had driven to the airport a hundred times.

I was panicking but trying to hide it. Was this what happens just before a heart attack ensues? The adrenaline was now pumping so furiously and frantically that I thought my chest would burst. I knew I would need to stay laser-focused to save us all from peril. "My life is not going to end on this highway in a fiery crash!" I vowed.

I guided my father with my trembling voice step-by-step, highway exit by highway exit, until we miraculously arrived at the airport terminal parking lot. At this point, he could not even recall how to use the parking entrance ticket machine. I exhaled.

The car came to a complete stop as my dad slumped over the steering wheel. Although my father's brain seemed to be completely shutting down, his spirit to get precious cargo—my mom and I—safely to our destination had kept his hands heroically on the wheel. Or perhaps he had passed the wheel to his guardian angels. I leapt from the car to get emergency assistance.

A few weeks later, my dad—my hero and biggest fan—would be diagnosed with stage IV brain cancer. His only warning signs had been migraine-like headaches and, of course, the odd lapse in memory.

From the outside, he presented as an extremely healthy six-foot-three, fifty-six-year-old man. The last place I thought I'd ever be hanging out with him was in the hospital waiting room for brain surgery patients.

After arduous surgery to remove my dad's brain tumor, the highly skilled yet emotionally unintelligent surgeon said, "I mucked around in there as long as I could, but I couldn't get it all—so he may never speak again."

Never speak again?

Those three words side-swiped me with the emotional impact of a Mack truck agonizingly crushing a subcompact car.

I leaned hard against the waiting room wall to keep from crumpling under the weight of this gut-wrenching news. Squeezing my mother's hand, I could not bear the look of anguish and helplessness in her tear-filled eyes.

At that moment, the mindset my dad had instilled in me—hopefulness and joy, risk-taking and optimism—drained from my soul. The tide had turned. I ceased to be a "twenty-something, bright-eyed, carefree, anything's-possible" daughter. I had no other choice than to be an "all-grown-up" emotional caretaker for my mom and dad.

In that moment, I vowed to myself: "For as long as it takes, I am going to become my best self for my parents." I decided to be the hardest-working, highest-achieving daughter possible. I knew I'd have to dig deep to find that place. Little did I know this was my intended journey all along, as painstakingly difficult as it would be.

After a year and a half of treatments and driving home every weekend to help my father learn to walk, write, and try to speak again, he succumbed to his disease. This was my first heart-wrenching grief experience—a dreadfully difficult loss—despite it being a great personal teacher. The "Cancer Club Family Alumni" membership I'd been gifted would continue to follow me for years to come. In fact, only a couple of years after my father's passing, my best friend's husband, Todd, was ironically diagnosed with the same inoperable brain tumor. Shortly thereafter, one of my closest work colleagues, Kathy, found out—while pregnant with twins—that she had stomach cancer. She was given less than a year to live. And then it was my turn to experience the Capital "F" Fear of a life-threatening tumor diagnosis.

Cancer Club

Cancer changes everything. It sucker-punches you, then pulls the rug out from under all of your hopes and dreams—everything you've known to be true. You become a member of the club no one wants to join, no one wants to talk about.

Barely thirty years old, I started my own merry-go-round journey of medical tests and specialist appointments. Eventually, I was referred to an Ear, Nose, and Throat doctor because I was having pain in my throat and chest. I would wake up in the middle of the night feeling like my left arm was completely paralyzed. It was terrifying. Specialist after specialist, X-ray after X-ray, no one could pin down the cause or the cure. Finally, a CAT scan and an MRI uncovered a lime-sized tumor on my first cervical rib. It had moved my trachea over an inch. The numbness in my arm and fingers now made perfect sense.

As a busy advertising executive in Montreal, I had to squeeze my medical appointments in between a full plate of client meetings. Detached and nonchalant, I remember walking into my appointment with the head surgeon at the Montreal Chest Institute, thinking it would simply be a quick chat about the laser surgery he'd perform to remove my "probably not cancerous" tumor. "Easy peasy," I thought to myself.

I was so wrong. Feeling alone and overwhelmed, I buckled under the gravity of the information the thoracic surgeon shared with me. I remember his words hitting me like a ton of bricks.

"Catherine, this is a very challenging surgery to perform, and the risks include paralysis on the left side of the body, optic nerve damage, and, of course, severed vocal cords." His words echoed throughout the room.

Just like my father's prognosis years earlier, I was being informed I may "never speak again." Ironically, I wanted to scream, but it felt as though I had no voice at all. No choice in the matter. Surgery was determined to be the only way to definitively know if my tumor was cancerous osteosarcoma or an osteochondroma (benign bony growth).

Either way, the surgeon expressed certainty that the tumor would eventually kill me, albeit painfully slowly. As if that's any consolation!

When my dad was diagnosed with a brain tumor, all I wanted was an answer to the questions, "Why is this happening to my amazing dad?" and "Why my happy family?" Now, here I was, asking, "Why ME?"

Everything that comes with a possible cancer diagnosis—family concerns, managing relationships, children, your job, your finances—can pull you down into a deep, dark abyss of uncertainty. Suddenly, the world can feel very, very bleak and unfair! And even for those who do not eventually receive a cancer diagnosis, their world is still profoundly, undeniably changed. That's because your brain receives news of "possible cancer" in the same way it processes a definitive cancer diagnosis—with dread, fear, and uncertainty. You're always on the lookout for the next dark package delivery, thinking maybe that one will be cancer. Maybe you cheated death this one time, but next time, you won't be so lucky.

It's a heavy symphony that keeps playing on repeat in a minor key—deeply embedded in your limbic brain.

You can never go back and pretend you didn't receive a wake-up call from the mortality gods. From that moment onward, your life is never the same. And even if you survive cancer and are given a clean slate, one question keeps swirling in your head: Is it really forever?

Capital "F" Fear keeps surreptitiously circling in the background, like spyware looking for its next victim.

My hunch is you've picked up this book because you're a part of the "Cancer Club" too. You're probably a lifetime card-carrying member by now with a platinum personal or family membership. Please know you're in good company no matter whether you arrived here as a caregiver, a survivor, or if you're currently awaiting lab results. Because even if the results come back as negative, a cancer ride is an extremely difficult, profound, life-altering experience. Please know that wherever you are, it's okay—you can navigate this journey at your own pace and in your own way.

In my case, I was convinced I was going to die from a cancer that had not even been confirmed. I had also decided that my dear mother would not suffer through the excruciatingly brutal experience of watching another loved one die a slow death. At that point in my young life, I'd had more than my share of experience with family and young friends dying of cancer. So why not me? As is often the case, declining physical health brings with it declining mental health. My rational brain became overwhelmed and clouded over with fatalistic, negative self-talk. I had no idea that I was suffering from severe clinical depression.

It was as if a freight train had crashed in my brain and knocked out all the power. I desperately needed to break free of this emotional train wreck and escape all the emotional pain.

So, at the height of this crippling emotional breakdown, I found myself teetering on the edge of the subway platform. Like many of the suicidal clients that I would help years later as a trauma therapist, I had no hope for a brighter future. All I wanted to do was escape the pain—just end it.

I am grateful that my best friend understood suicidal ideation and drove through the night to get me the medical intervention I desperately needed. The long climb out of this dark hole was an arduous process. But with antidepressant medication that rebooted my biochemistry, cognitive behavioral therapy to tackle my self-sabotaging thoughts, and supportive family and friends, my depression started to lift.

A few months later, I was ready to choose whether to have the risky thoracic surgery or to play a waiting game. I chose the surgery. I soldiered on. And for all intents and purposes, the surgery was a resounding success.

Shortly after the lab analysis confirmed that my tumor was the benign, non-cancerous kind, I received a phone call from my dear friend and work colleague, Kathy. She was the friend who found out, while pregnant with twins, that she had terminal stomach cancer. Kathy had delivered two healthy baby boys and was busy writing journals and making time capsules for their future life milestones. What an unbelievably heart-wrenching situation. I've never felt so guilty in my life—telling someone I did not have cancer—as I did with Kathy that day.

I could feel her spirit beaming on the other end of the phone as she said, "I'm so happy you have good news, Cath. There's so much you're meant to do in this lifetime. You're such a bright light."

Cancer Awakening: Self-Surrender and Why We Need It

So there I was, on the wide-open roadway of life, paralyzed by the enormity of my good fortune, unable to reconcile why a mother of twins would have her life cut short while I was allowed to live. That day marked the beginning of my spiritual awakening—breaking free of negative patterns and emotional pain—a lifelong mental health resiliency roadway I'm still on today.

It was almost as though I'd been given the freedom to climb inside my box of darkness, bitterness, and grief. Permission to emerge with a whole new sense of self. Permission to start edging along the pathway toward self-acceptance and self-enjoyment again. To be honest, I was learning to practice self-surrender for the first time ever; something I endeavored to consciously practice every day thereafter.

Let's face it: sooner or later, we all receive some news that brings us to our knees and rocks our very foundation. It may be news of something that has been brewing for a long time, such as terminal cancer, or it may be a sudden event like a terrible car accident. Either way, it can push us to our limit.

What I can tell you from my own life experience and from working with hundreds of clients is that self-surrender is one of the best coping tools available to you right now. Surrender happens when you no longer believe or think you have all the answers. You remain hopeful but without all the struggle.

You can't continue to operate as before. The game is up. You can't control the future or produce a guaranteed result. So, you learn to let go and release everything to a higher power beyond the thinking mind.

That's ultimately a good thing because self-surrender focuses your attention on the present moment like never before—the here and now. You relinquish control, which is necessary for living life with more ease, more joy, and less striving. Self-surrender happens when you throw out your old GPS and trust that this new boat will carry you wherever you need to go. Paradoxically, when you embrace *not* knowing where your cancer journey might lead, you tap into a higher self-knowing or deep well of insight.

*Mindfulness is one of the best boats I know of
to get you across that churning river of fear.*

Although we can't just snap our fingers and decide to cultivate mindfulness, practicing gratitude is an easy way to start shifting your focus from worrying about the future to acknowledging what you're grateful for in the present. Research has shown that one positive, thankful interaction every morning has the power to set your entire day on a more positive path. Several scientific journals, including the *Journal of Positive Psychology*, have reported that mindfulness and gratitude are linked to better mental and physical health, self-awareness, better relationships, an overall enhanced sense of fulfillment, and a decrease in pain. (N. Swain, B. Lennox Thompson, S Gallagher, J. Paddison & S Mercer [2020] Gratitude Enhanced Mindfulness [GEM]: A pilot study of an internet-delivered programme for self-management of pain and disability in people with arthritis, The Journal of Positive Psychology, 15:3, 420-426, DOI: 10.1080/17439760.2019.1627397)

* * *

For one week, I challenge you to take a few moments at the end of each day to reflect, acknowledge, and write down three things you are grateful for and why. Consider keeping a beautiful gratitude journal by your bedside. Instead of focusing your attention on what you've lost on your cancer journey, be grateful for this "cancer awakening" and all the goodness in your life. Some families practice gratitude as they sit down for a meal at the kitchen table. Others see gratitude as a form of prayer, pausing to give thanks for simple blessings. We have a choice to live today, viewing everything we're grateful for as a gift.

* * *

Over time, I have learned that self-surrender and self-enjoyment can also be found in all of the quiet little twinkly moments—petting your dog, tickling a child, smelling the lilac blooms, holding your lover's hand, or feeling a warm breeze. It's a very personal experience of living—the sheer pleasure of being alive that vibrates in each of us.

Spiritual Leader Michael Beckwith, in an episode of Oprah's *Super*

Soul Sunday podcast, remarked, "We're not in this world to get anything—we are in this world to let something unfold from within us."

I encourage you to marvel at each of the hardships and cancer diagnoses you've survived so far. The traumas you survived when you thought you might not.

You did survive. AND you've kept on surviving. How amazing is that?!

It's our struggles, past and present, that sow the seeds for authentic growth and resiliency.

It's not about striving, desperately seeking answers, or doing something to fix it. It's not one more thing on your "to-do" list or something you need to get over. It's simply the dark package that's landed on your doorstep today, this month, this year. It's acknowledging BEING—simply breathing. Breathing in the relief of just letting go. It's "human being" versus "human doing" that's been reprogrammed in our brains.

I'd also like to acknowledge that whether you're a cancer survivor, a cancer caretaker, or that hypervigilant "I think I have cancer" person, there is light in your dark journey. The light is often obscured by the big "F" of FEAR, but it does exist. It's buried in the bottom of that deep, dark package. And it's okay if you can't see it or even conceive of it right now. Maybe you never will. That's okay, too.

Cancer gives us the opportunity to be with profound anguish—perhaps for the first time ever. The chance to fully experience the fury and get all in that puddle of pain. It forces you to walk a lonely, painful path home to yourself. As a survivor and seasoned trauma therapist, the one thing I know to be true is: "You have to feel it all to heal it all."

This experience has also been called "the dark night of the soul," a term rooted in medieval Christianity used to describe the mental breakdown that many mystics experienced prior to a spiritual awakening. When you stumble upon your own "unfolding" or "awakening", there will be no disguising it.

And yes, there's a gift inside for those who choose to see it that way.

Cancer Gifts

The wound is the place where the light enters you.
—*Rumi*

I'd love to sit down beside you, give you a giant hug, and remind you once again that there's light in this dark package called cancer. As a trauma therapist, I also know that everyone's suffering is different. Until you have a possible cancer diagnosis you can never know what your process will be. Nothing I can say is going to make this go away or get you across the bridge faster.

The only way through it is through it.

Yes, it's hard; it takes the time it takes, and the process for each human being is unique. Yet, even though most people don't come with the software or algorithm to cope, I've seen people fully flourish after a cancer diagnosis. I've also witnessed a father who had lost everything because of cancer embrace deeper love for his children and experience joy beyond anything he had ever known before. Ultimately, as adults, we can choose how to apply our minds and our spirits and reach out for community or cultural resources that will support this kind of healing and growth.

I also believe cancer can be a dark gift that helps us evolve, thrive, and foster what is known as post-traumatic growth (PTG).

This is a fancy term for a phenomenon psychologists have been studying over the past twenty-five years. It describes how negative experiences really can result in positive change, including newfound personal strengths, improved relationships, a deeper appreciation for life, spiritual growth, and exploration of new possibilities. Many people have reported that they experience a stronger sense of self because of having endured a period of great adversity, like surviving cancer.

So, PTG is the dark gift—the struggle to reconstruct our lives after our worldview and conditioned beliefs have been shattered. This dark gift can lead to shifting priorities and pivotal changes that may greatly benefit both your life and the lives of many others. *Post-traumatic growth is probably what helped you bounce back from your last traumatic experience. And it's the gift to be opened in your current cancer ride.*

Gleaned from fifteen years of studying survivors of trauma, Dr. Martin E. P. Seligman, founder of positive psychology, identified the single most important trait for post-traumatic growth: "learned optimism." He noted that survivors with an optimistic attitude say things like "I'm not giving up"; "This setback is temporary and changeable"; "It's just this one situation"; and "I can do something about it."

Perhaps the best antidote to traumatic change is "tragic optimism," a phrase coined by the existential-humanistic psychologist and Holocaust survivor Viktor Frankl. Tragic optimism refers to the ability to find meaning and purpose amid the inevitable tragedies of our human existence instead of being crushed or overwhelmed by them.

I give thanks every day for my tumor and the post-traumatic growth I experienced as a result. After completing my disability leave post-surgery, I could not return to my job as an advertising executive, selling cough syrup to babies and creating new versions of laundry detergent. I had crossed the bridge to self-actualization and joined the indomitable "cancer club."

You can never go back to your old way of life after such a profoundly transformative experience. Just like a butterfly emerging from a chrysalis, traumatic change is often the difficult catalyst to realize our amazing potential—our true gifts.

As much as I loved my advertising agency job, I realized that I could no longer work in an industry focused on frivolity and mind-numbing consumerism. I needed to do something more socially redeeming than creating commercials for products people really didn't need. I was motivated and inspired to make a difference in the world. I needed to be in a helping profession.

So, I contacted the psychology departments of two different universities to determine the psychology course prerequisites I would need to apply for a Master's degree in Counselling Psychology. I requested letters of support from one of my old university professors, from a former boss, and from the doctor who first investigated my tumor (and supported me throughout my entire medical journey).

Holding my Master's degree in my hands three years later was one of the proudest moments of my life. For the past twenty-five years, I have had the honor of helping a wide range of individuals move beyond crippling emotional darkness to find their own light.

If someone had asked me years ago, "What could you do for hours on end, never get bored, and feel completely fulfilled?" I would have answered, "Talking to people, trying to figure out their motivations, helping them rise above adversity, and writing good news stories."

I've indeed found my North Star—my contribution that adds value to the world and holds great value for me as a mental health educator, inspirational speaker, and now best-selling author. I believe whatever you're passionate about—your life legacy—is patiently waiting for you to emerge from the darkness that is cancer, too.

* * *

Here are three simple steps to uncover your own post-traumatic growth:

- **Step 1:** Start by naming, writing down, or describing out loud your current cancer ride—the dark package—in your life.
- **Step 2:** Say "thank you" for the feelings this adversity triggers, such as fear, sadness, or envy. Breathe.
- **Step 3:** Write down or think about what this experience has taught you so far about yourself that you otherwise would never have known.

Now ask yourself the following questions:

- How has this dark package motivated me to change my behavior and evolve for the better? Am I motivated to serve my highest good and help others as a result?

- What role did self-surrender or mindfulness play? Have you had a spiritual awakening or transformation? Describe it. Did you develop a deeper relationship or a new skill or strength as a result?
- In what way is this experience worthy of your gratitude now? Take a moment to name it. "I'm grateful for _____." Breathe in gratitude. Place your hand on your heart. Smile.

* * *

Cancer Hero

Hard times don't create heroes.
It is during the hard times when the 'hero' within us is revealed.
—Bob Riley

Every day, I think about how fortunate I am to be on this Earth, how fortunate I am to see the sunrise and experience another day. As a cancer club member, you are your own special breed of hero. It takes great courage to face your greatest fears—stare down death—and keep moving forward. On the cancer roadway, you must endure bumpy patches, emotional upheaval, physical pain, and way too many life detours to even count. It's not easy to surrender everything you've ever known to be true, leave behind old ways of being, and start completely anew.

Let's think about this cancer road trip as your own personal Hero's Journey—the journey from suffering to enlightenment that spiritual leaders have described for centuries; the same series of experiences that Joseph Campbell outlined in his 1949 book, *The Hero with a Thousand Faces,* that every individual goes through—whether you're Mother Teresa, Luke Skywalker, or amazing you.

Being a cancer hero means you get back up on your Hero's Journey. You live. You learn. You choose a new route. You slay your dragons. What choice do you have when you're literally sideswiped by a dark package?

Resilience in the face of cancer is not about heroically toughing it out alone.

Reaching out to friends and community members for support, advice, and encouragement along the roadway is also vital to overcoming adversity and coping well with cancer. Having a strong network of supportive family and friends just might save your life. I'm only here today because my oldest and dearest friend, Laurie, literally thwarted my suicide plan.

In closing this chapter, let's validate and honor how resilient you already are—what you've survived. Look at the trials and tribulations you've faced—the dark packages—on your wild cancer ride. There's growth to be found in all our challenges that enables us to move through them and find the gift of transformation that our souls are seeking.

You are already a hero. You are already more than enough. You have resiliency deep within your bones, and there's no time like the present to lift the lid and bring it all up to the surface. Let's stop chasing "enough" and finally accept that we already have all that we need to thrive on this cancer quest.

I'd also like to remind you that you've survived one hundred percent of all your very worst days. *You're still here.* Searing hardships like cancer gives us the opportunity to better understand ourselves, our worldview, and our relationships. Perhaps more than anything else, they literally propel us toward a new mindset and new life pathway. It takes enormous courage to get to the other side of this struggle. Some days, that courage may simply involve getting out of bed in the morning. But persistence and perseverance after repeated falls will demonstrate your extraordinary capacity to rise—your heroic nature.

Psychologist Dr. Angela Duckworth coined the idea of "grit" to describe people who are highly resilient in the face of life's challenges—true heroes. Being gritty is being able to push yourself through difficult circumstances, finding a way above, below, or around an obstacle, temporarily failing while consistently moving toward a passionate goal. If the key attribute of a resilient person is optimism, then the salient attribute of a gritty person is a sustained, never-give-up attitude when working toward achieving a goal. And we sure as heck need the grit to have grace under fire when confronted with a cancer diagnosis.

* * *

Here are a few ways to learn how to build this mindset while you navigate the difficult path ahead:

1. Interview someone who has experienced a tragedy like terminal cancer and lived to tell the tale—what helped them through it?
2. Find examples of grit in nature. Think about how you can be more like a tulip bulb or a tree sprouting in the rubble of a junkyard.
3. Embrace problems or mistakes as temporary setbacks and opportunities to grow and change.
4. Decide that everything is "figureoutable" if you break a problem down into bite-sized, manageable pieces and set mini-goals for your day.
5. Heraclitus said, "The only constant in life is change." Sometimes, a goal needs to be abandoned because it is no longer attainable. Practice self-compassion. Repeat the *Serenity Prayer*, and fully surrender to forces beyond your control.
6. Practice observing the parts of your cancer journey that might be funny or quirky. Laugh at yourself at least three times today. Remember whatever is happening will probably make a funny— albeit darkly humorous—story one day.

* * *

It is my hope that you will continue to welcome the wisdom in your dark packages—the pain, the detours, the epiphanies, and the rejection—along the cancer roadway. Painful experiences will always be part of my life and yours, but the mark of a purposeful life is how we accept, embrace, and unwrap these dark packages and then graciously gift them to the world. Taking ownership allows us to evolve pain into empowerment, transmute suffering into strength, and transform loss into opportunity. **You are a Cancer Hero just for showing up here today!**

I've interviewed and portrayed people who've withstood some of the ugliest things life can throw at you, but the one quality all of them seem to share is an ability to maintain hope for a brighter morning—even during our darkest nights.
—Oprah Winfrey

CATHERINE CLARK

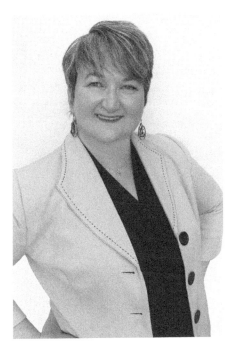

Catherine Clark, MEd, is a Certified Canadian Counsellor, award-winning speaker, best-selling author, and owner of Catherine Clark Connects (*catherineclarkconnects.com*), a boutique mental health consulting firm in Toronto, Canada.

Catherine is passionate about creating psychologically safe workplaces and reducing the stigma of mental illness. Over the past twenty-five years, she has trained thousands of adult learners and C-suite executives, equipping them with coping tools to thrive personally and professionally. She has worked with the Inuit and Dene populations in the Canadian Arctic, Francophone agencies in Montreal, and a wide range of multinational corporations across North America.

In her first book, *Gifts in Dark Packages*—written during the pandemic—Catherine offers readers a roadmap to resiliency and good mental health by harnessing the power of adversity. She shares her own personal downward spiral in life as well as relatable case studies to illustrate how using these actions can channel adversity into resiliency, propelling people forward and helping them emerge from difficult times to live life with greater joy and ease. A work-life balance advocate, Catherine enjoys decompressing in nature and being a purveyor of the arts. Her greatest love is sharing laughter with her two "twenty-something" children.

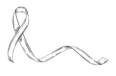

ACKNOWLEDGMENTS

I am deeply grateful for the incredible support I have received as I prepared to launch this book into the world. It takes a whole village to raise a child—and to nurture any vision. I knew this book could come to life with the support of a village of steadfast, strong women. However, I did not anticipate that this village would propel my vision for this project beyond the limits of my own imagination. For this, I am eternally grateful.

I extend a heartfelt thank-you to each author and Cancer Hero in this book. I greatly appreciate your unique gifts and profound contributions to my life and this literary project. I love, honor, and celebrate each one of you! A giant thanks for believing in my dreams and trusting in me.

I am grateful to my editor and publisher, Jennifer Goulden of Entourage, for her magical way of taking my idea and bringing this beautiful book to fruition. Thank you for melding together the words in this book with your tears and rewriting them with so much love and sensitivity. Many hearts are beating in sync to serve the world through this book, and your heart plays the lead note.

To my film crew, Amreen Ghouse, Kamraan Mohammed, and Will Bink, thank you for bringing the authors' stories to life in such a poignant and captivating way. I greatly appreciate how you filmed each author with tears in your eyes—listening to and capturing each storyteller with your whole heart.

To my friend, Gaby Mammone, you are my "Google heart!" I cannot thank you enough for your knowledge, insight, kindness, unconditional love, encouragement, and support.

To my Coach, Dwania Peele, for your powerful stand for me and my visions. You make things happen!

To all the co-authors, Catherine Clark, LaCountess Ingram, Niki Papaioannou, Pat Labez, Rowena Rodriguez, Shirley Gaudon, Tania Kolar, and CoCo Roper, YOU ARE EXTRAORDINARY. It has been an honor to see you share a glimpse of your greatness in this book. Your presence is a contribution to the world. Thank you for trusting me with your personal life experiences and for sharing your stories so generously. Catherine, Niki, and Tania, thank you for supporting me with your expertise as team players.

To my four beautiful children, Simrah, Ashaz, Ruby, and Sarah, thank you for being kind and patient with me and giving me the space needed to put this book together. You sacrificed several hours of "mommy and you" time for me to complete this project. I am deeply honored by your generosity, love, and support.

Thank you to my parents for choosing to provide me with a good education. I am especially grateful to my mother for instilling in me the discipline needed to be a lifelong learner.

Lastly, I am grateful to Matt Thorne for his beautiful heart—the way he loves and cares deeply for the world. Your mother is a Cancer Hero, and her greatness lives in you. There is hope because there is you.

HONOR A CANCER HERO IN YOUR LIFE

To add the name of a Cancer Hero (you or a loved one) to the next edition of Cancer Heroes and to have the authors write you or your loved one's name on a ribbon as part of our tapestry, visit

www.cancerherostories.com

READ MORE

To make a donation or to see updates on Cancer Heroes, their stories, events, and news, visit us online:

CANCER HEROES

Cancer Heroes are all around us.
Here, we are honoring those who are experiencing cancer or who have in the past.

Margaret Hough

Edwin Arnold

Jack Arnold

Doris Thomson

Jayanth Das

Sakina Ariff

Sultana Tikari

Andrew Shackleton

Peter Dennett

Andrew Dennett

Ruthe Martin

Angela Irwin

Carl Steinman

Bill Ingram

Queen Esther Ingram

Louis Ingram

Nikia Jefferson

Wanda A. Williams

Miriam Wright-Nesbitt

Cynthia Wright

Judy Ketchen

Doreen Bierman

Tracy Weber

Joyce Schefold

Derek Schefold

Lolly Murray

Dieter Herkert

Jan Strassburger

Estelle Strassberger

Kristine Williams

Shirley Thum

Vivian Gibson

Gary Morton

Amynmohamed Harji

Samantha Willacy

Michelle Kauntz

Rick Steenkist

Each of the names above will be written on a ribbon and woven into the Cancer Heroes tapestry. To add a name of a Cancer Hero in your life: *cancerherostories.com*

Made in the USA
Middletown, DE
10 May 2024